Perspectives on Medical Research
Volume 2, 1990

Edited by

Stephen R. Kaufman, M.D.
Kathryn Hahner, Ph.D.
Joan Dunayer

Published by the Medical Research Modernization Committee

Published by
Medical Research Modernization Committee

Printed in the United States of America

For information, contact the Medical Research Modernization Committee, Box 6036 Grand Central Station, New York, NY 10163-6018.

Library of Congress National Serials Data Program
International Standard Serial Number 1053-8984

ISBN 0-9623858-0-8
ISBN 0-9623858-1-6 (pbk)

Editorial Board

Contents

Essays

Animal Models of Spinal Cord Injury
Stephen R. Kaufman, M.D. 1

The Relationship between Laboratory and Clinical Studies in Psychopharmacologic Discovery
Brandon P. Reines, D.V.M. 13

Spheroid Cultures for Cancer Research and Treatment
Ron Allison, M.D. 27

Review of Scoliosis Research at the University of Michigan
Joel D. Mack, M.D., Robert A. Greenberg, M.D. 33

Debunking Myths in Nursing Theory and Research
Peggy L. Chinn, R.N., Ph.D., F.A.A.N. 37

Baby Fae: The Unlearned Lesson
Kenneth P. Stoller, M.D. 49

NIH Research Protocol for Silver Spring Monkeys: A Case of Scientific Misconduct
Neal D. Barnard, M.D., Roy Selby, M.D., Daniel T. Robinson, Ph.D., Gervasia M. Schreckenberg, Ph.D., Carol Van Petten, M.D. 52

Evaluation of Bone Graft Research
Neal D. Barnard, M.D. 93

Book Reviews 97

C.F.M. Hendriksen: *Laboratory Animals in Vaccine Production and Control*
Reviewed by Ron Allison

Gill Langley (Ed.): *Animal Experimentation: The Consensus Changes*
Reviewed by Kathryn Hahner

Alan M. Goldberg (Ed.): *In Vitro Toxicology: New Directions*
Reviewed by Paul Contard

Bernard E. Rollin: *The Unheeded Cry: Animal Consciousness, Animal Pain and Science*
Reviewed by Eric Dunayer

Preface

Because *Perspectives* has become the primary publication of the Medical Research Modernization Committee, it is important that the monograph's scope correspond to that of the MRMC. While the reliability of animal research has been a leading concern of the MRMC, it is not the only subject of interest. Some of the issue's essays deal with topics of little, if any, relevance to the animal research controversy. They address strengths and weaknesses of different research strategies, reflecting the MRMC's goal of evaluating a broad range of research approaches in order to identify and promote the most efficient and reliable methodologies. Consequently, our annual monograph series, previously titled *Perspectives on Animal Research*, will now be titled *Perspectives on Medical Research*, which better describes the purview of both the MRMC and this publication.

In this volume, Peggy Chinn exposes underlying assumptions of the traditional medical scientific method. She proposes that nursing research employ an alternative approach, called "future search," to enhance knowledge and human well-being. Ron Allison reviews a new and exciting *in vitro* technology known as spheroid cultures. Their clinical value remains unproven, but their potential includes strategies to individualize cancer therapy. Kenneth Stoller investigates legal and moral issues surrounding the much-publicized Baby Fae case. Offering evidence that Baby Fae's rights were violated, Stoller raises concerns about the ability of either the scientific community or the general public to protect the rights of vulnerable human research subjects.

Brandon Reines continues his ongoing survey of the historical role of animal research in medical discovery. Rejecting the traditional view that animal models have led the process of psychiatric drug discovery, he advocates increased postmarket surveillance of drugs in order to note side-effects that suggest new therapeutic applications for those drugs.

Neal Barnard and colleagues review the case of the Silver Spring Monkeys. They present evidence that research protocols advocated by highly placed government officials were not designed to advance medical science, but to kill animals whose history has become a considerable public relations burden for the research community. Information presented in the article indicates that leaders in the scientific community acted out of improper motives and permitted public relations to take precedence over good science. In another article, Barnard criticizes a protocol to test a new bone-graft substance on greyhounds. He points out how the animal model fails to reproduce critical elements of traumatic bone damage.

As in the first volume of this series, several articles critically review animal models of human diseases. Stephen Kaufman challenges the clinical relevance of animal models of spinal cord injury and discusses problems inherent in animal models of human diseases. Similarly, Mack and Greenberg find that an experimental model of scoliosis does not relate meaningfully to the human counterpart.

A new feature of this volume is the inclusion of advertisements. It is the policy of *Perspectives on Medical Research* that all advertisements be printed free of charge, to keep editorial policy uninfluenced by advertisers. The advertisements are included to inform our readers of publications they may find of interest.

Biographical Information on the Contributors

Neal D. Barnard, M.D.

Dr. Barnard is a practicing physician and President of the Physicians Committee for Responsible Medicine. He is a graduate of the George Washington University School of Medicine and completed a residency in psychiatry at the same institution. He is certified by the American Board of Psychiatry and Neurology.

Peggy L. Chinn, Ph.D.

Dr. Chinn received her Ph.D. in Educational Psychology from the University of Utah. She is a Fellow of the American Academy of Nursing, the author of several texts, and editor of *Advances in Nursing Science*. She has been actively engaged in health-related research for more than 20 years, and she is currently Professor of Nursing and Director of Graduate Programs at the University of Colorado Health Sciences Center School of Nursing.

Robert A. Greenberg, M.D., M.S.P.H.

Dr. Greenberg received his A.B. from Harvard College, M.D. from the University of Pennsylvania, and M.S.P.H. in epidemiology from the University of North Carolin at Chapel Hill. He completed a residency in pediatrics at the Children's Hospital Medical Center in Boston and is certified by the American Board of Pediatrics. For the past 20 years, he has practiced and taught pediatrics as a full time faculty member of the University of North Carolina at Chapel Hill.

Stephen R. Kaufman, M.D.

Dr. Kaufman received a B.A. from Yale University and an M.D. from Case Western Reserve University. He completed an ophthalmology residency at New York University Medical Center. He is currently a retina fellow at Manhattan Eye Ear & Throat Hospital. He was the principal investigator of a review of animal models of human diseases, published as Volume 1 supplement of *Perspectives on Animal Research*. He is the Vice-Chair of the Medical Research Modernization Committee.

Joel D. Mack, M.D., F.A.C.S.

Dr. Mack received an A.B. from Harvard College and an M.D. from Harvard Medical School. He did general surgery and orthopedic residency training at the University of Minnesota Hospitals, and he is certified by the American Board of Orthopedic Surgery. He is in private orthopedic practice, and he is Vice Chairman of the Board of the Greater Bakersfield Memorial Hospital.

Carol Van Petten, M.D.

Dr. Van Petten received her M.D. degree at the University of Wisconsin and completed residency in neurology at the University of Southern California. She is currently a fellow at the Neuromuscular Center of the University of Southern California.

Brandon P. Reines, D.V.M.

Dr. Reines received a B.S. from the University of Massachusetts and a D.V.M. from Tufts University. He is Director of The Center for Health Science Policy in Arlington, Virginia. His monographs include *Cancer Research on Animals: Impact and Alternatives*, *Heart Research on Animals: A Critique of Animal Models of Cardiovascular Disease*, *Psychology Experiments on Animals: A Critique of Animal Models of Human Psychopathology*, and *Environmental Experiments on Animals: A Critique of Animal Models of Heatstroke, Frostbite, and Hypoxemia.*

Daniel N. Robinson, Ph.D.

Dr. Robinson is Professor and Chairman of the Department of Psychology at Georgetown University, Washington, D.C. He received his doctorate in Neuropsychology from the City University of New York and is the author of numerous texts and articles on human perception and brain function.

Gervasia M. Schreckenberg, Ph.D.

Dr. Schreckenberg is Professor of Neurobiology at Georgian Court College, New Jersey. Dr. Schreckenberg received her Ph.D. from the Catholic University, Washington, D.C., and completed post-doctoral training at Columbia University. She was previously on the biology faculties of Fairleigh Dickinson University and the University of Texas at Austin.

Roy Selby, M.D.

Dr. Selby is the former Chairman of Neurosurgery at Cook County Hospital, Chicago, Illinois. Dr. Selby is a graduate of the University of Arkansas School of Medicine. He completed residency at the Veterans Administration Hospital, Little Rock Arkansas and University of Illinois Neuropsychiatric Institute. His fellowship was at the Lehey Clinic in Boston, Massachusetts.

Kenneth P. Stoller, M.D.

Dr. Stoller was an undergraduate at the University of California at Los Angeles, where he was a University of California Presidents Undergraduate Fellow. He received his postgraduate training at the U.C.L.A. Department of Pediatrics. He is a Fellow of the American Academy of Pediatrics. He is Board Certified in pediatrics, and he is currently in pediatric private practice. He has published papers in a wide range of fields, including pediatric infectious disease, eye movement, and remote physiological sensing.

Correction

Kathryn Hahner's credentials were listed incorrectly in Volume 1. Dr. Hahner is a licensed psychologist whose Ph.D. is in Social/Personality Psychology.

Animal Models of Spinal Cord Injury

Stephen R. Kaufman, M.D.

Introduction

There are approximately 7,000 new cases of paraplegia or quadriplegia annually as a consequence of traumatic spinal cord injury (SCI), making SCI a leading cause of disability in the United States. Many cases of SCI are either too severe for any hope of functional recovery or mild enough to permit symptoms to resolve spontaneously. The remaining patients might benefit from medical intervention to minimize the effect of the acute injury and/or reduce the damage from later secondary effects of trauma. There has been extensive research in an effort to develop animal models that might yield insights into the nature of SCI and help guide treatment strategies. However, in attempting to create a standardized, reproducible spinal cord injury in animals, researchers use highly artificial, unnatural injuries that do not appear to relate meaningfully to human SCI.

Experimental SCI

Early experimental spinal cord injuries involved dropping animals from heights or hitting animals on the back with a board.[1] In 1911, Allen reported a new technique that allowed much more precise quantification and standardization of injury.[2] Allen first removed soft tissues and vertebral bone; then he dropped weights through a tube positioned directly on the exposed spinal cord. Later modifications included use of an "impounder" at the base of the tube to distribute the forces more precisely and techniques to stabilize the rest of the spinal column. This impact model is used most widely today, and cats are the most common experimental subjects. Other techniques of SCI, such as compression by a balloon,[3] are also employed.

Problems with the Impact Model

Maiman has suggested the following criteria for evaluating the soundness of an SCI model: "First of all, a spinal cord injury model should be physiologic: that is, it should accurately reproduce the anatomic and functional changes seen in clinical injury. Second, it must be both quantifiable and reproducible, so that effects of modifying agents can be determined."[5]

Experimental SCI does resemble clinical SCI in the gross neurological deficits seen, but there are fundamental pathological differences between the two conditions. Maiman has noted that SCI induced by the direct impact model typically produces central hemorrhage in the spinal cord and that such hemorrhage is rare in human patients:

> Among the best studies of the histologic changes seen in SCI are those published by Kakulas. In patients dying within 24 hours after SCI, cord lacerations, as well as subarachnoid and epidural hemorrhage, were common. In contradistinction to much of the experimental literature based on the dorsal impact model, significant hematomyelia (blood in the spinal cord) was rarely seen; in addition, microscopic/neuronal changes were uncommon. . . . Necrosis, but no gross hemorrhage, was common in the central grey matter.[4]

Work by Ducker and Hamit reveals further discrepancies between experimental and clinical SCI. Ducker and Hamit found that a force equivalent to a firm tap, when directly applied to the spine, was sufficient to paralyze almost 100% of dogs.[5] In contrast, while human SCI victims generally experience forceful trauma to the back, these forces are distributed by soft tissues and bone. Removing these tissues creates an artificial condition that does not necessarily reflect the actual forces upon the spinal cord in human SCI. As Maiman notes, "Varying amounts of delivered forces are absorbed in the bone or disc, or they may be effectively transmitted to the spinal cord. Certainly, it is not unusual to see severe fractures with minimal cord injury, and vice versa."[4] In addition, the impact model fails to address traction forces due to angulation of the spine during injury.[4]

Furthermore, the localized impact of this model is quite uncommon in human SCI, in which several spinal segments are usually damaged.[4] "Variations in lesion length," Blight has noted, "may be of prime importance for functional outcome. This problem has not been addressed at all, yet it is one of the most striking differences between animal models and human injuries."[6]

Similarly, in animal models the injury is restricted to the spinal cord, while in humans vertebral bone injuries are common. In a large clinical study, Bracken et al. reported that over half the patients had spinal fractures and dislocations; over 40% had bone fragments.[7] Experimental SCI fails to account for these factors.

Although experimental SCI has been directed toward creating reproducible injuries, results have not been uniform. Findings based on animal studies have retained considerable variability. In the impact model, Hitchon et al. found, the size of the spinal cord, its elasticity, and the extent of laminectomy all influenced injury outcome.[8] Ford has commented, "Animals with apparently identical threshold injuries inflicted by Allen's technique do not all become permanently paraplegic, nor does the histological appearance of their chronically injured cords consistently relate to functional recovery."[9]

Extensive efforts to control experimental SCI have so far failed. Blight notes:

> We have taken a number of simple precautions to control for gross physical variables. The first of these was to stabilize the spinal cord against a solid base. This can be done by introducing a metal hook under the cord, but we chose to use the vertebra itself as an "anvil" to avoid additional manipulation of the cord. This was done by separating the rib articulations and passing steel supports under the transverse processes of the vertebra below the impact site. This simplifies the mechanics of impact by removing the reaction of the thorax and the stiffness of surrounding vertebral articulations as variables. . . . Residual variations in the biomechanics of the cord . . . are less easily dealt with. They include the resting tension in the elastic elements, the tissue fluid pressure, the blood pressure, the relative diameters of the cord and the vertebral canal, the relation of the impact site to nerve roots and pial blood vessels. In addition, if we are to use as an endpoint the number of axons that survive, we should take into account the variation in the number and density of axons in the cord before injury, as well as the approximations implicit in our measurement of them. When these elements are added together, their contribution to the overall variability of outcome is likely to outweigh the approximations involved in generating or calculating the mechanical impulse delivered by a simple weight drop.[6]

Collins, too, cites problematic variability:

> Physiological factors that alter blood flow or metabolism, alter outcome, and the minimal controls in any experimental spinal cord injury model must include body temperature, blood pressure, PO_2, PCO_2, and blood pH. Many studies have failed to consider these controls and entered variables that make interpretations of the result difficult to impossible.[10]

Another problem with the impact model is the use of laminectomy.[11] Albin and White have criticized this aspect of the model: By "exposing the spinal cord to infection and other cellular changes" and "removing the anatomical energy-attenuating structures (e.g., hair, skin, bone, and muscle mass) so that a relatively small amount of force can produce major damage," laminectomy leads to "lack of correlation with pathologic changes found in the human; inability to study biomechanical factors concerning vertebral body, posterior elements and ligaments; and variability in lesion development resulting from the differences in design of weight-dropping systems."[12]

Laminectomy also artificially alters blood flow to the spinal cord. In the bone surgery of laminectomy, it is necessary to ligate or cauterize many vessels. Given that it is widely believed that spinal cord ischemia is largely responsible for secondary damage to the injured spinal cord, laminectomy's alteration of normal blood flow should arouse concern. Nevertheless, in my review of the literature, I did not encounter any discussion of this issue by laboratory or clinical researchers.

Recognizing the difficulty of controlling injury in the impact models, Hitchon et al. have suggested that compression of the spinal cord with a balloon might create a more reproducible injury. The balloon compresses the cord for periods of five minutes ("acute" injury) to several hours. Clearly, this differs from the instantaneous damage that occurs in the clinical SCI setting.[10] Hitchon et al. have acknowledged:

> It is difficult to believe that any apparatus used for the study of cord compression can serve to mimic cord injury as encountered in our medical practice. The latter injuries may be secondary to a multitude of compressive, angular or distraction forces. Clinically encountered injuries are complex, and thus their duplication in the laboratory with one particular method is literally impossible.[8]

Problems with Using Animal Models to Assess SCI Progression

"Postmortem material from acute cases has revealed some useful facts about the nature of severe injury, but does not tell us about pathophysiology or the condition of the surviving population," Blight has noted in defense of animal models.[6] However, just as autopsies require the patient's death, animal subjects are killed for pathological examination. Consequently, in an individual animal, the progression of the pathological process cannot be histologically studied. Theoretically, this problem is resolved by giving many animals identical injuries, which can then be studied at different time intervals. In reality, however, there are difficulties in controlling SCI experimentally, and there is considerable anatomical variability even among individuals of a single species.[6] Even if these variables could be controlled, the artificial nature of the experimental injury makes its clinical applicability tenuous. In contrast, the progression of SCI in humans can be reliably studied by performing autopsies on patients who have died at different intervals after injury.

The Failure of Animal Models to Uncover Effective Therapies

Maiman has observed, "In the last two decades, at least 22 agents have been found to be therapeutic in experimental SCI . . .. Unfortunately, to date none of these has been proved effective in clinical SCI."[4] This poor correlation between laboratory and clinical findings with regard to drugs' therapeutic potential is likely due to the experimental injury's artificiality. For example, many clinicians believe that edema plays a role in human SCI[13]; yet, laminectomy may reduce some of the damage due to edema.[14] Consequently, the standard impact model may not accurately reflect the post-injury changes that contribute to secondary damage in human SCI patients.

There are several possible explanations for the discrepancies between the animal and human data.[14] As noted by Janssen and Hansebout, animals are given injuries of moderate severity, in order to highlight any effect of a drug treatment. In contrast, as mentioned earlier, most human injuries are either too severe for any therapy to help or so mild that recovery occurs without treatment.[14] Also, newer treatments tend to be reserved for the most extreme cases that have little likelihood of improvement. These factors have made it difficult to validate, in patients, any treatment suggested by animal studies. Janssen and Hansebout have also observed:

> Experimental SCI often involves a carefully controlled and directed blow or compression to a single portion of the cord under sterile conditions and only after anesthetic has been given and vital functions reinforced. The human injury, conversely, is often associated with injuries to internal organs, loss of blood, and introduction of foreign material into the blood and tissues leading to infections, shock, emotional distress, etc.[14]

Conflicting results have further impeded efforts to interpret the experimental literature. Use of different models, commencement of therapy at different times, and, in studies of drug treatment, use of different dosage sizes and schedules can contribute to the inconsistency of laboratory results. Albin and White have noted the inconsistent value of many therapeutic modalities, including spinal cord hypothermia, naloxone, and corticosteroids.[14]

Use of Methylprednisolone in Human SCI

In 1990, the second National Acute Spinal Cord Injury Study (NASCIS

2) demonstrated that a short course of "megadose" methylprednisolone (a corticosteroid) was beneficial in acute SCI.[7] NASCIS 1, conducted with a different dosage regimen, had not shown benefit from methylprednisolone.[15] The NASCIS 2 report, as well as a commentary in the same issue of the *New England Journal of Medicine*, credited the animal model with revealing the efficacy of this dosage of medication.[16] This claim was not justified.

Although megadose (30 mg/kg) steroid treatment has been efficacious in both animal tests and human clinical trials, the animal data did not predict the human results.

First, the NASCIS 1 study did not rule out the possible efficacy of *lower* steroid doses. This study compared a bolus of 100 mg methylprednisolone followed by ten daily infusions of 100 mg methylprednisolone to a 1000 mg bolus followed by the same ten day regimen of 100 mg of the steroid. The study found no significant difference between the two treatment groups.[15] Because there was no control group that received placebo, it is possible that *both* regimens were efficacious.

Second, the animal data also did not rule out the efficacy of lower steroid doses. While many animal model systems have shown a benefit from high dose steroids approximating those of the NASCIS 2 study,[17-24] many also indicated that lower doses were efficacious.[25-27] Therefore, the animal model data did not demonstrate that megadose steroids were necessary.

Third, while most animal studies have shown a beneficial effect from steroids, there have been conflicting reports on the value of steroids.[12,28] Several investigators studying low dose steroids,[29,30] high dose steroids[31] and both doses[32] have found no clinical benefit from this therapy. Those who claim that the animal data predicted the human findings are ignoring the fact that the animal data are inconsistent.

Fourth, the dosage regimen in the animal studies differed from that in the clinical study. The human patients received the first dose, a bolus dose, an average of 8.7 $\pm$ 3.0 hours after injury. In contrast, the experimental animals received their first dose much sooner. I was able to locate seven of the eight animal research articles cited by Ducker that "better defined the appropriate dose."[16] All the experimental subjects in these papers received their first steroid dose 30-60 minutes after injury.[18-24] Having found that 30 mg/kg methylprednisolone given 4 1/2 hours after experimental injury was ineffective, Hall et al. concluded, "It would appear that the ability of the steroid to reverse the ischemia once it has developed is limited, and probably lost, within a few hours of onset."[27] Therefore, contrary to the claims of Bracken et al.,[7] Ducker,[16] and others,[33,34] the animal data actually indicated that the

NASCIS 2 clinical trial would fail.

Fifth, the animal studies were unnecessary precursors to clinical studies, because clinicians had good reasons to expect steroids to be helpful in treating human SCI. Indeed, five years after the NASCIS 1 report, Janssen and Hansebout wrote that, although the efficacy of steroids in treating SCI "remains unsettled, many physicians still elect to treat with steroids as soon as possible after injury."[14] Furthermore, *high-dose* steroids have been used safely and effectively in the management of head trauma[35] and edema of nervous tissue[36] for decades. There was little doubt, then, that high-dose steroids would also be safe in treating SCI, and there was good reason to believe that they would be efficacious. The expectation of safety and the good possibility of efficacy, in fact, is the reason that NASCIS 1 did not include a control (placebo) group. The NASCIS 1 protocol reflected the belief of the investigators that it would be unethical to deny SCI patients steroid treatment.[16]

Sixth, many promising experimental results have not been useful clinically. As mentioned above, Maiman noted in 1988 that none of the 22 agents found to be therapeutic experimentally has been proven efficacious clinically. Indeed, NASCIS 2 had a naloxone treatment arm, based in part on encouraging laboratory results. Patients receiving naloxone, however, did not benefit from this treatment.[7] In calling attention to the alleged contribution of animal studies toward the development of one SCI treatment (high-dose methylprednisolone), researchers ignore the fact that the vast majority of animal studies have failed to lead to successful treatments.

Problems with Animal Models in General

It appears that, at best, clinical researchers learn about human SCI and then, *in retrospect*, note which animal models appear to support their conclusions. Nevertheless, Hitchon et al. have written that "these animal models are invaluable, for each allows us to study one particular facet of cord injury, but definitely not the entire spectrum of spinal injuries."[8] This comment reflects a widespread tenet among animal researchers that each discovery about one aspect of a disease helps elucidate the entire disease process. This belief is based on a faith in the validity of "reductionist" methodologies -- employed in almost every animal-based biomedical research project.

The underlying assumption of reductionism is that an entire process can be understood as the sum of its individual parts. Reductionist thinking is conducive to laboratory science, in which researchers attempt to control all variables except one, manipulate that variable, and draw conclusions about its nature. For example, researchers have used different amounts of impact force in experimental SCI in order to evaluate the effect of different forces on spinal cord damage.

There are, however, at least two problems with reductionist methodologies in experimental SCI. First, in an effort to control all other variables, the researchers induce an injury that corresponds poorly to human SCI. Spinal cord damage due to trauma reflects more than the impact of force on the spinal cord. It also reflects such factors as interaction of the spinal cord with damaged soft tissue and bone, trauma-induced changes in systemic blood pressure, and changes in vascular tone. In the experimental setting, all of these factors are altered, in an effort to control variables. These interventions create artifacts that make interpretation of the research difficult. Second, this reductionist approach fails to account for the interactions among different organ systems that are altered by SCI. In the human clinical setting, SCI induces changes in the systemic circulation, the immune system, the musculoskeletal system, and other bodily functions, as well as the spinal cord. These changes in the circulatory, immune, central nervous, and other systems interact with one another. Consequently, reductionist experimental SCI does not provide valid information about human SCI.

In general, information derived from a "model" that is fundamentally different from any human condition may be quantitative, reproducible, and statistically significant, but its relevance is limited to the artificial laboratory condition. It is exceedingly unlikely that such research will be useful for the management of any human disease.

Alternatives to Experimental SCI

The search for greater understanding and improved treatment of human SCI will require research. Given that the animal model is a poor analogue to human SCI, progress will most likely require use of a range of human clinical investigative tools. For example, observations of the natural histories of different human injuries will yield insights into SCI's pathological processes. Every SCI case represents an "experiment of Nature."[37-39] Each offers insights into SCI's causes and consequences. The value of clinical material is enhanced by non-invasive imaging technologies, such as CAT, MRI, and PET scans, which can be useful in evaluating anatomical and metabolic changes after neurological trauma.[40,41] Also, a vast amount of pathological material is available on autopsy. Because many SCI victims die hours or days after injury, the consequences of SCI can also be studied at different points in time.[42] In addition, the mechanical forces that injure spinal tissue can be evaluated quatitatively by subjecting human cadavers to forces commonly experienced during trauma.[43]

The prospective, randomized clinical trial, such as that of NASCIS 2,[7] is currently the "gold standard" methodology in determining optimal therapy. Experimental SCI has not been very useful in identifying promising therapies to be evaluated by such studies. In contrast, clinical experience is a valuable source of information. The value of steroids in the management of cerebral edema, for example, has encouraged many clinicians to use steroids in an effort to minimize damage after SCI.

Clinical serendipity, which has been critical to major advances in other fields,[44-46] may yield new discoveries. For example, it is possible that some patients given a medication to treat damage to organs other than the spinal cord may recover neurologically to a surprising degree. This could stimulate a carefully controlled clinical trial to determine if that medication really were helpful in the SCI setting. Thorough reporting of medications and outcomes of all SCI patients, facilitated by the availability of inexpensive computers, would increase the likelihood that serendipitous insights could be exploited.

Also, recently developed technologies have facilitated the study of neurological tissues *in vitro*.[47-49] *In vitro* techniques could help identify drugs that minimize damage due to cellular changes after trauma.

Conclusion

There has been extensive use of experimental SCI, but the value of this research is undemonstrated. The animal model, which differs from human SCI in many fundamental respects, has a poor track record in identifying useful treatments of human SCI.

If experimental SCI is of minimal relevance to our understanding and treatment of human SCI, why do many scientists endorse the experimental model so strongly? One reason is financial incentive. The unnatural conditions of experimental SCI are said to yield "new" and "interesting" results -- thereby stimulating generous research support. Funding does not, however, signify that animal research is scientifically or medically useful.

References

1. Dohrmann GJ: Experimental spinal cord trauma: A historical review. *Arch Neurol* 1972;27:468-473.
2. Allen AR: Surgery of experimental lesion of spinal cord equivalent to crush injury of fracture dislocation of spinal column: A preliminary report. *JAMA* 1911;57:878-880.
3. Tarlov IM, Klinger H, Vitale S: Spinal cord compression studies: Experimental techniques to produce acute and gradual compression. *Arch Neurol and Psych* 1953;70:813-819.
4. Maiman D: Symposium on spinal cord injury models: Introduction. *J Am Paraplegia Soc* 1988;11:23-25.
5. Ducker TB, Hamit HF: Experimental treatments of acute spinal cord injury. *J Neurosurg* 1969;30:693-697.
6. Blight A: Mechanical factors in experimental spinal cord injury. *J Am Paraplegia Soc* 1988;11:26-34.
7. Bracken MB, Shepard MJ, Collins WF, et al.: A randomized, controlled trial of methylprednisolone or naloxone in the treatment of acute spinal-cord injury. *N Engl J Med* 1990;322:1405-1411.
8. Hitchon PW, Lobosky JM, Wilkinson TT, Dyste GN, Girton RA: Impact and balloon compression models of the spinal cord. *J Am Paraplegia Soc* 1988;11:35-40.
9. Ford RWJ: A reproducible spinal cord injury model in the cat. *J Neurosurg* 1983;59: 268-275.
10. Collins WF: A review and update of experimental and clinical studies of spinal cord injury. *Paraplegia* 1983;21:204-219.
11. Koozekanani SH, Vise WM, Hashemi RM, McGhee RB: Possible mechanisms for observed pathophysiological variability in experimental spinal cord injury by the method of Allen. *J Neurosurg* 1976;44:429-434.
12. Albin MS, White RJ: Epidemiology, physiopathology, and experimental therapeutics of acute spinal cord injury. *Crit Care Clin* 1987;3:441-452.
13. Weiss MH: Mid- and lower cervical spinal injuries, in Wilkins RH, Rengachary SS (eds): *Neurosurgery*, New York, McGraw-Hill, 1985.
14. Janssen L, Hansebout RR: Pathology of spinal cord injury and new treatments: A review. *Spine* 1989;14:23-32.
15. Bracken MB, Collins WF, Freeman DF, et al.: Efficacy of methylprednisolone in acute spinal cord injury. *JAMA* 1984;251:45-52.
16. Ducker TB: Treatment of spinal cord injury. *N Engl J Med* 1990;322:1459-1461.
17. Green BA, Kahn T, Klose KJ: A comparative study of steroid therapy in acute experimental spinal cord injury. *Surg Neurol* 1980;13:91-97.
18. Means ED, Anderson DK, Waters TR, Kalaf L: Effects of methylprednisolone in compression trauma to the feline spinal cord. *J Neurosurg* 1981;55:200-208.
19. Anderson DK, Means ED, Waters TR, Green ES: Microvascular perfusion and metabolism in injured spinal cord after methylprednisolone treatment. *J Neurosurg* 1982;56:106-113.
20. Braughler JM, Hall ED: Correlation of methylprednisolone levels in cat spinal cord with its effects on (NA^+ + K^+)-ATPase, lipid peroxidation, and alpha motor neuron function. *J Neurosurg* 1982;56:838-844.

21. Young W, Flamm ES: Effect of high-dose corticosteroid therapy on blood flow, evoked potentials, and extracellular calcium in experimental spinal injury. *J Neurosurg* 1982;57:667-673.
22. Hall ED, Wolf DL, Braughler JM: Effects of a single large dose of methylprednisolone sodium succinate on posttraumatic spinal cord ischemia: Dose response and time-action analysis. *J Neurosurg* 1984;61:124-130.
23. Braughler JM, Hall ED: Effects of multi-dose methylprednisolone sodium succinate administration on injured cat spinal cord neurofilament degradation and energy metabolism. *J Neurosurg* 1984;61:290-295.
24. Braughler JM, Hall ED, Means ED, Waters TR, Anderson DK: Evaluation of an intensive methylprednisolone sodium succinate dosage regimen in experimental spinal cord injury. *J Neurosurg* 1987;67:102-105.
25. Ducker TB, Hamit HF: Experimental treatments of acute spinal cord injury. *J Neurosurg* 1969;30:693-697.
26. Lewin MG, Hansebout RR, Pappius HM: Chemical characteristics of traumatic spinal cord edema in cats. Effects of steroids on potassium depletion. *J Neurosurg* 1974;40:65-75.
27. Kuchner EF, Hansebout RR: Combined steroid and hypothermia treatment of experimental spinal cord injury. *Surg Neurol* 1976;6:371-376.
28. Hall ED, Braughler JM: Glucocorticoid mechanisms in acute spinal cord injury: A review and therapeutic rationale. *Surg Neurol* 1982;18:320-327.
29. Faden AI, Jacobs TP, Holaday JW: Thyrotropin-releasing hormone improves neurologic recovery after spinal trauma in cats. *N Eng J Med* 1981;305:1063-1067.
30. Rucker NC, Lumb WV, Scott RJ: Combined pharmacologic and surgical treatments for acute spinal cord trauma. *Am J Vet Res* 1981;42:1138-1142.
31. Hedeman LS, Sil R: Studies in experimental spinal cord trauma. Part 2: Comparison of treatment with steroids, low molecular weight dextran, and catecholamine blockade. *J Neurosurg* 1974;40:44-51.
32. Eidelberg E, Staten E, Watkins CJ, Smith JS: Treatment of experimental spinal cord injury in ferrets. *Surg Neurol* 1976;6:243-246.
33. Flamm ES: How animal research has helped. *Philadelphia Inquirer*, April 23, 1990.
34. Loeb JM, Runkle DC: Responding to the animal activists. *Issues in Science and Technology* 1990;6(4):31-34.
35. French LA: The use of steroids in the treatment of cerebral edema. *Bull NY Acad Med* 1966;42:301-311.
36. Galicich JH, French LA: Use of dexamethasone in the treatment of cerebral edema resulting from brain tumors and brain surgery. *Amer Practitioner* 1961;12:169-174.
37. Reines BP: On the role of clinical anomaly in Harvey's discovery of the mechanism of the pulse. *Perspec Biol Med*, in press.
38. McQuarrie I: *The Experiments of Nature and Other Essays*. Lawrence, KS, Univ Kansas, 1944.
39. Humphreys W: *Anomalies and Scientific Theories*. San Francisco, Freeman, Cooper, and Co, 1968.
40. Djang WT: Radiology of acute spinal cord trauma. *Crit Care Clin* 1987;3:495-518.
41. Quencer RM: The injured spinal cord: Evaluation with magnetic resonance and intraoperative sonography. *Radiol Clin North Amer* 1988;26:1025-1045.

42. Kakulas BA, Jacobsen PF, Bedbrook GM: Acute spinal injuries. A Clinicopathologic study. *Proc 19th Veterans Admin Cord Injury Conf*, Scottsdale, Arizona, 1973, pp 84-95.
43. Yoganandan N, Sances A, Maiman DJ, Myklebust JB, Pech P, Larson SJ: Experimental spinal injuries with vertical impact. *Spine* 1986;11:855-860.
44. Reines BP: The rationale for postmarketing surveillance as a means of drug discovery for mental illness. *Perspec An Res*, in press.
45. Good RA: Runestones in immunology. *J Immunol* 1976;1176:1413-1428.
46. Good RA: Keystones. *J Clin Invest* 1968;47:1466-1471.
47. Alliot F, Pessac B: Astrocytic cell clones derived from established cultures of 8-day postnatal mouse cerebella. *Brain Res* 1984;306:283-291.
48. Cepko C: Immortalization of neural cells via oncogene transduction. *Trends Neurosci* 1988;11:6-8.
49. Ronnett GV, Hester LD, Nye JS, Connors K, Snyder SH: Human cortical neuronal cell line: Establishment from a patient with unilateral megalencephaly. *Science* 1990;248: 603-605.

Psychopharmacologic Discovery: The Relative Contributions of Clinical and Laboratory Studies

Brandon P. Reines, D.V.M.

Discovery of the modern antipsychotic and antidepressant drugs did not, as many believe, begin with laboratory investigations; it evolved throughout the 19th century, as organic chemists observed the effects of synthesized carbon compounds on the human central nervous system (CNS). McIlwain has written, "Last century's application of synthetic organic chemicals in medicine can be viewed as an experiment, lasting several generations and contemporaneous with the development of organic syntheses themselves, in which animals and men were exposed to all the main categories of the newly produced chemicals. . . . The main groups of synthetic drugs in fact all acted on the brain [i.e., affected awareness]."[1]

The discoverers of modern psychopharmacology were clinical investigators who noted mood-altering side-effects of drugs used in clinical practice. Drugs administered for therapeutic purposes often induce unforeseen alterations in human physiology and/or cognition. Physicians who note these alterations are in an ideal position to identify and explain clinical anomalies caused by pharmacological intervention. Many of pharmacology's "lead" compounds, including the psychiatric medications, were discovered in the clinical context.

Phenothiazine Tranquilizers

The discovery of chlorpromazine's antipsychotic action evolved during the 1930s, 1940s, and 1950s, based on the mood-altering side-effects of its predecessors, the antihistamines. In the late 1930s, such dicyclic antihistamines as phenbenzamine, diphenhydramine, and mepyramine were in wide clinical use. The antihistamines' most striking clinical side-effect was CNS depression -- drowsiness.[2] In the late 1930s, P. Charpentier had synthesized the first tricyclic antihistamine, promethazine, which had a strong sedative effect. She then synthesized a variety of promethazine analogues, including chlorpromazine. In the early 1950s, the French surgeon H. Laborit, aware of the antihistamines' central-depressant effects, undertook a search for an antihistamine to use as a preanesthetic sedative. Charpentier sent chlorpromazine to Laborit to test as a preanesthetic sedative based on the antihistamines' known CNS depressant effects and the results of animal tests, in particular the mouse pole-climbing test.

When Laborit first administered chlorpromazine to his surgical patients, he was stunned by its effect on the human CNS. The patients seemed to become totally indifferent to their surroundings, experiencing what Laborit called "euphoric quietude."[2] As a result, Laborit persuaded his psychiatric colleagues to test chlorpromazine on psychotic patients. Chlorpromazine developed into the first major antipsychotic because clinical application of the drug as a presurgical sedative caused physicians to notice its mood-altering side-effects.

In a recent A.M.A.-sponsored book, F.D. Campion claims that chlorpromazine was discovered by experiments on rodents.[3] Campion has written:

> In the early 1950's researchers in France who were testing a phenothiazine compound . . . observed some remarkable behavior in the mice they were using. These had been psychologically conditioned, much in the manner of Pavlov's dog, to climb a pole in their cage in response to the sound of a buzzer. The conditioning had been done by sending a sharp jolt of electricity through the floor of their cage at the moment the buzzer sounded.
>
> Having been conditioned, the mice then received doses of phenothiazine. Now when subjected to the electrical charge, the mice would still scamper up the pole. But no longer would they do so merely in response to the buzzer. It was apparent that the phenothiazine acted selectively: it could depress the nervous system of the mice sufficiently to quiet the conditioned reflexes while leaving the psychomotor reactions unimpaired.
>
> On the strength of this finding, the drug was tried on an institutionalized psychotic with such astounding results that he was discharged three weeks later.

The claim is misleading on a number of counts. First, phenothiazines were not tested on animals for behavioral effects *until* Laborit had identified the clinical phenomenon of phenothiazine-induced ataraxia. Campion misrepresents the discovery of chlorpromazine's antipsychotic properties as an "accidental" laboratory discovery. Reines[4] argues that provivisection propagandists, in order to secure priority of discovery for laboratory studies, often misrepresent the process of medical discovery as a fortuitous consequence of accidental laboratory findings. In fact, the theory that chlorpromazine would prove an effective antipsychotic was deduced from Laborit's clinical observations -- not animal experiments. Second, most of the early animal behavior experiments failed to reproduce the calming effect Laborit had seen in his patients.[5] Third, the selection of chlorpromazine was based on results of an animal test researchers considered useful in identifying a superior preanesthetic sedative, not an effective antipsychotic. Finally, the pole-climbing test was uninterpretable. Apart from the difficulty of extrapolating from one species to another, the test results did not necessarily reflect sedation. The drug's effect on the mice might have been, instead, balance impairment, loss of muscular tone, apathy induction, or some other physiological or psychological alteration. It was Laborit who recognized chlorpromazine's potential as an antipsychotic. At most, the pole-climbing experiment dramatized Laborit's clinical hypothesis that phenothiazines have profound effects on the human CNS.

Tricyclic Antidepressants, Benzodiazepines, and Dibenzodiazepines

While lithium and the monoamine oxidase inhibitors were discovered serendipitously, many other psychotropic drugs, including the tricyclic antidepressants, benzodiazepines, dibenzodiazepines, and other neuroleptics evolved out of the work on chlorpromazine. The structures of these psychotropics were "deduced" from chlorpromazine's structure. (Fig. 1-3) The phenothiazines, tricyclic antidepressants, and dibenzodiazepines are all tricyclics. Along with the benzodiazepines, they are all congeners of chlorpromazine. In fact, the scientists who synthesized the tricyclic antidepressants and the benzodiazepines have acknowledged being inspired by chlorpromazine's structure.[6]

Indeed, the tricyclic antidepressants were originally developed as antipsychotics. During clinical trials, however, R. Kuhn found that their primary effect was CNS stimulation rather than depression. That observation led Kuhn to test the tricyclic imipramine as an antidepressant.[7] Sulser and Mishra have written:

> It was the discovery by Delay and Deniker [following Laborit's work] in France of the unusual therapeutic value of chlorpromazine in the treatment of psychosis that revived clinical research interests in the structurally related iminodibenzyl compounds [tricyclic antidepressants]. The similarities in pharmacological properties of chlorpromazine and some of the iminodibenzyl derivates prompted Roland Kuhn, at the Psychiatric Clinic in Munsterlingen, Switzerland, to test some of these new compounds synthesized by the Geigy chemists as potential antipsychotic agents in patients with various psychiatric disorders, including endogenous depression. . . . Further clinical studies with another compound of this series that was structurally more similar to chlorpromazine . . . now known to be imipramine . . . resulted in the unexpected discovery of the therapeutic value of imipramine in the treatment of endogenous depression.[8]

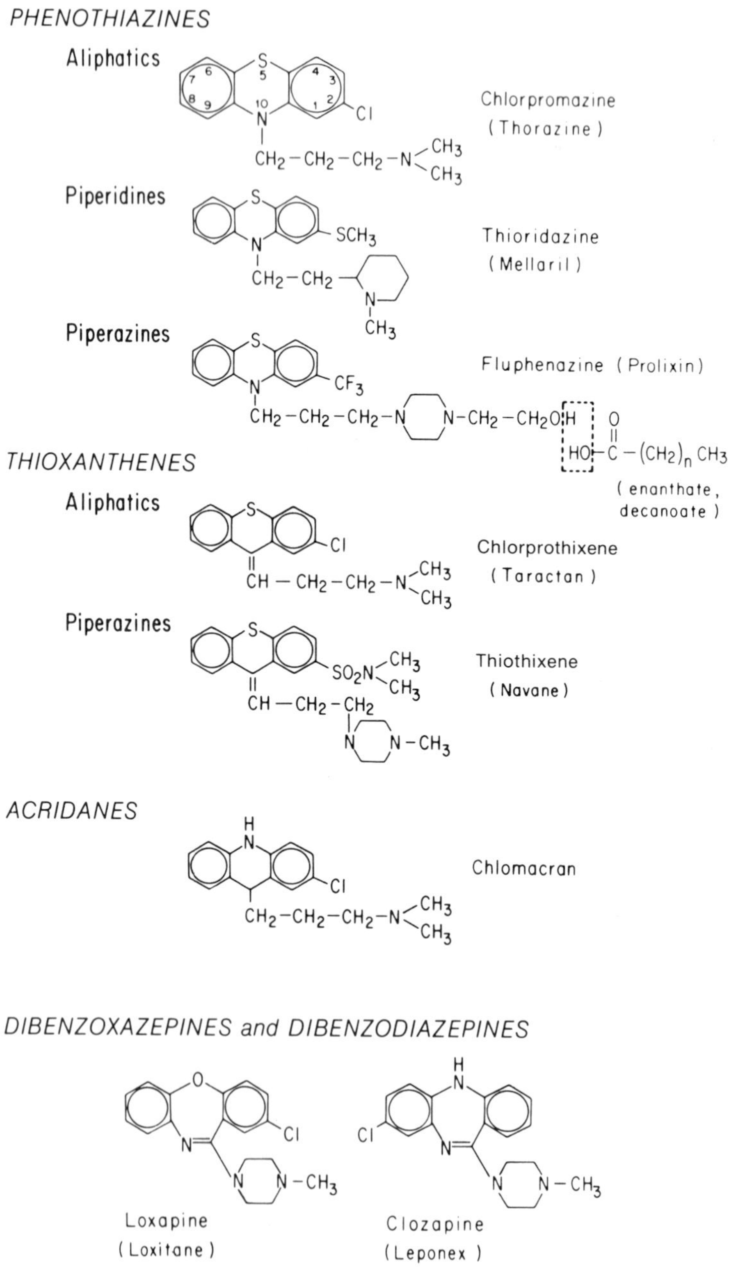

Figure 1. Tricyclic antipsychotic agents.

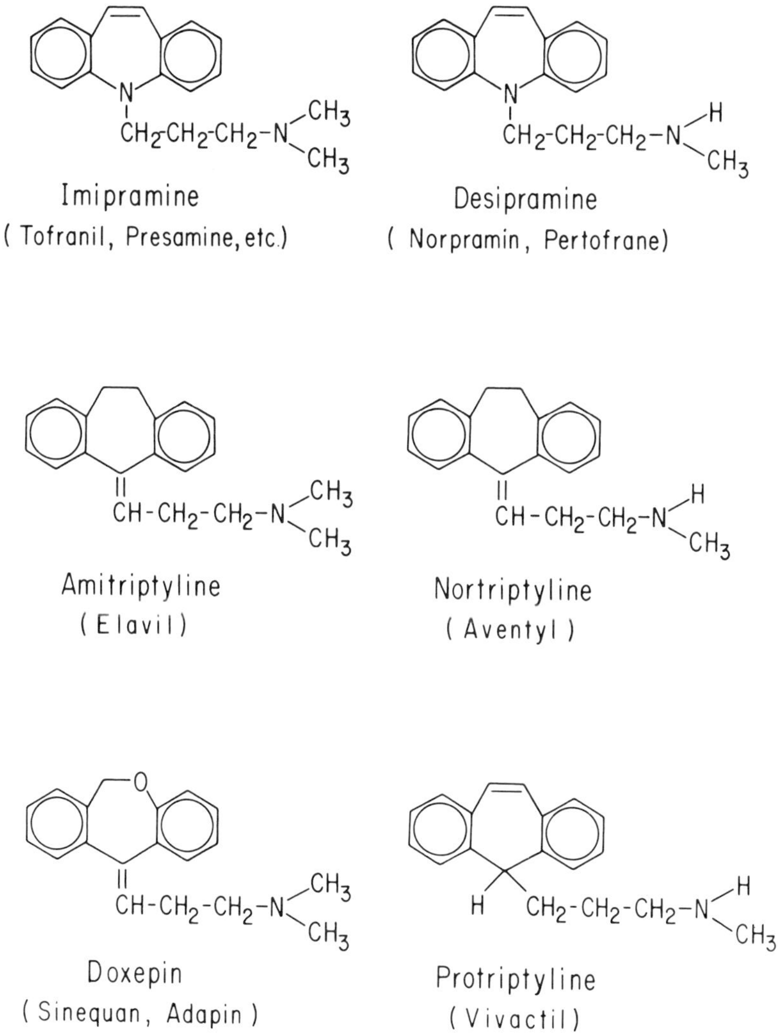

Figure 5. Tricyclic antidepressants.

SEDATIVE-ANTIANXIETY AGENTS

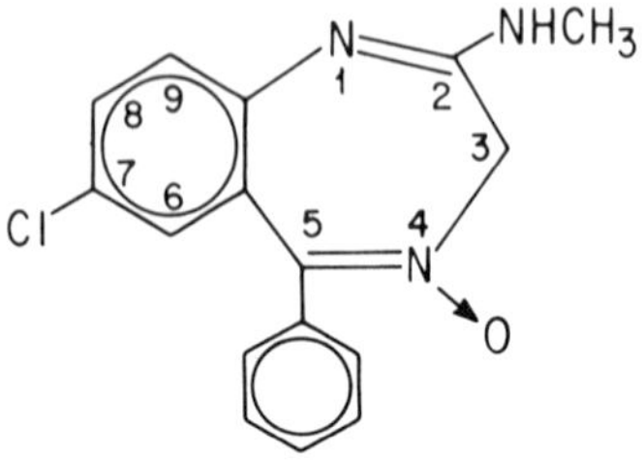

Chlordiazepoxide
(Librium)

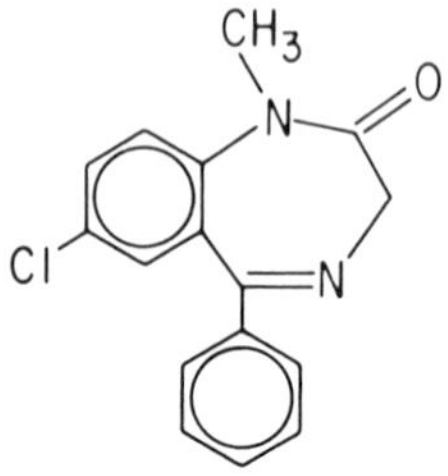

Diazepam
(Valium)

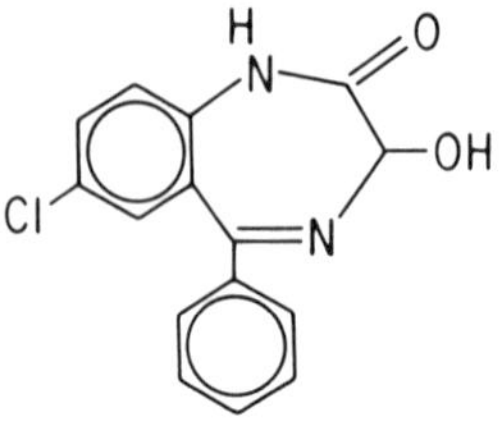

Oxazepam
(Serax)

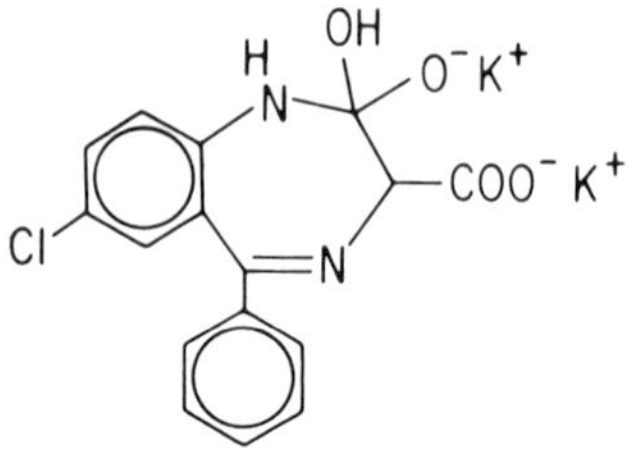

Chlorazepate
(Tranxene)

SEDATIVE-HYPNOTICS

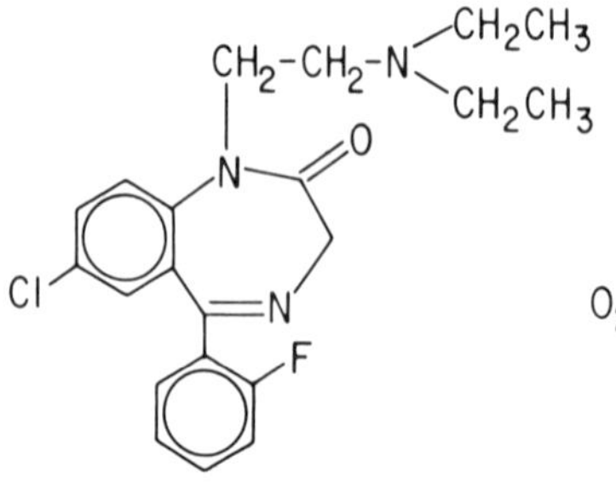

Flurazepam
(Dalmane)

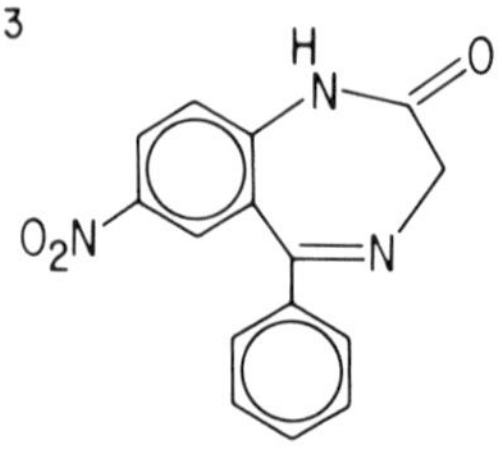

Nitrazepam
(Mogodon)

Figure 9. Benzodiazepine sedative-tranquilizers and hypnotics

Kuhn did not perform animal behavior studies to convince his colleagues of imipramine's potential efficacy in combatting endogenous depression. He was able to convince other psychiatrists based on clinical data alone.

Dr. E. Sternbach's synthesis of the first benzodiazepines was also inspired by chlorpromazine's tricyclic structure, on which he patterned the dicyclic structure of chlordiazepoxide (Librium) and diazepam (Valium).[6] The compounds were tested for efficacy on animals rendered artificially aggressive by experimental manipulations. According to W. Haefly, the compounds' "taming effect," particularly in "vicious cynomolgus monkeys," especially impressed pharmacologists.[9] The relationship between experimental aggression and human anxiety, however, is not at all clear. Although animal experiments were often used to dramatize the clinical potential of chlorpromazine's various analogues, dramatic impact should not be equated with scientific content. It was Laborit's, Kuhn's, and Sternbach's clinical hypotheses that ushered in the era of modern antipsychotic, antidepressant, and anxiolytic chemotherapy.

Monoamine Oxidase (MAO) Inhibitors

MAO inhibitors' antidepressant effect, like that of the dicyclic and tricyclic compounds, was discovered in humans. N.S. Kline, who was intimately involved with the discovery, recalls iproniazid's side-effect of "euphoria" in tuberculosis patients:

> Iproniazid had been introduced some years earlier as an experimental treatment for tuberculosis. . . . As a side effect, however, there developed an odd problem. The patients felt too good. They overexerted themselves and generally ignored the medical safeguards their condition required. Iproniazid's potential as a mood drug had gone largely unnoticed because psychiatrists at the time just weren't thinking along those lines. As the climate changed, however, a few researchers began to investigate it in a tentative way.[10]

Kline had good reason to expect iproniazid to have mood-elevating properties. Prior to clinical studies on depressed patients, he had reviewed the literature and found that, for unclear reasons, iproniazid had been clinically tested as a tranquilizer (i.e., CNS depressant). Not surprisingly, iproniazid had failed as a tranquilizer. Kline had ample clinical evidence to justify a clinical trial of iproniazid as an antidepressant, but he first used animal results in an intriguing way to convince his colleagues.

In early 1956, pharmacologists had used iproniazid on reserpine-treated animals in order to prevent reserpine's calming effects. This research was inspired by the knowledge that iproniazid elevated the mood of human tuberculosis patients. The animals did become hyperactive upon iproniazid administration; the results, however, were ambiguous. Lehman and Kline have reported that they were uncertain as to what was causing the "anti-depressant" effect: "We were not sure at first whether the animal results were due primarily to iproniazid (Marsilid) or to the Marsilid-reserpine combination and so we tried both approaches. In due course, we found that Marsilid alone could achieve the desired psychic energizing effect [in animals], and thereafter we concentrated the research on the use of the single drug."[10] This expressed uncertainty is odd, given that Kline was well aware -- long before 1956 animal tests -- that reserpine is a human tranquilizer, not a mood-elevating substance. In fact, he had already helped introduce reserpine into clinical use as a tranquilizer. Apparently, Kline was also aware of iproniazid's mood-elevating effects in humans. The available clinical data, therefore, were sufficient to lead Kline and his co-workers to theorize that iproniazid would be an effective antidepressant in patients. Evidently, the animal studies were performed to convince members of the hospital staff that the clinical data on iproniazid's effects were accurate. In any case, Kline's contention that the animal experiments showed that "Marsilid alone could achieve the desired psychic energizing effect" is simply false. Iproniazid's "psychic energizing effect" could not be evaluated with animal experiments because subtle psychic phenomena can only be studied in humans.

Lithium

In a recent paean to animal behavior studies, Pincus et al. maintained, "It is essential to recognize the vital importance of research use of animals to progress in psychiatric practice and knowledge. . . . Lithium, a drug whose clinical potential was first suggested by animal experiments, has dramatically benefitted hundreds of thousands of manic-depressive patients."[11] Similarly, in *Newsday*, F. Goodwin of ADAMHA claimed that experiments on guinea pigs led to discovery of lithium's antimanic action.[12] Goodwin did not discuss the origin of the main antipsychotics and antidepressants, presumably because psychopharmacologists know that these were discovered in the clinical setting and that the lead compounds would not have been detected by the common animal behavior tests.[13] In contrast, few psychopharmacologists know how lithium's antimanic effects were discovered. The drug's "clinical potential" was *not* "first suggested by animal experiments."

Discovery of lithium's antimanic properties is generally attributed to laboratory studies. In 1949, Australian physician John Cade injected guinea pigs with lithium ion. Rapidly, the guinea pigs became unresponsive to stimuli. Generations of historians have assumed that Cade's guinea pigs were rendered inactive by lithium's calming effect. Kline,[14] however, has argued that the guinea pigs were likely poisoned by the lithium. The fact that there are such varied interpretations testifies to the impossibility of studying subtle psychic phenomena in nonhuman animals.

Reines[4] argues that Cade's interpretation of his guinea pig results were biased by his knowledge of 19th century clinical literature indicating lithium's mood-altering properties.[13] Lithium caused depression among patients who were being treated for various conditions, such as gout.[15] In fact, the drug was used to treat various mood disorders, such as depression and "gouty mania," in the 1880s and 1890s.[16,17] Cade even reviewed lithium's CNS-depressant side-effects in the introduction to his classic paper.[18] Nevertheless, many modern pharmacologists either are unaware of or choose to ignore the older clinical literature. Discovery of lithium's antimanic action fits the historical pattern: Lithium's mood-altering side-effects were first identified in humans.

Bupropion

Is the recent discovery of the antidepressant bupropion an exception to the rule of clinical discovery? Bupropion, structurally unrelated to other antidepressants and antipsychotics, has been touted by some investigators as a triumph of animal modelling.[19] However, the drug's initial chemical structure was based, in part, on the structure of drugs that tend to confer sympathomimetic properties.[20] Sympathomimetics, such as amphetamine, are well-known CNS stimulants. Indeed, there is evidence that bupropion's development was inspired by the structure of amphetamine,[21,22] which had been used, with limited success, as an antidepressant in the 1930s.[23,24]

In order to ensure that the FDA would permit clinical trials, however, bupropion's manufacturers tested it for efficacy on a series of animal models of depression. Interestingly, the widely used tetrabenazine suppression test was not encouraging. (Tetrabenazine is a reserpine analogue.) Bupropion had a relatively low potency compared to other antidepressants. Also, unlike most antidepressants, bupropion, at peak effect, conferred less than 50%

antagonism of tetrabenazine.[25] Bupropion passed the L-dopa potentiation test, but Cooper et al. acknowledge that this test "has been shown to produce a relatively large number of false positive responses."[25] Finally, bupropion was encouraging in the "behavioral despair model" that tests a drug's ability to relieve immobilization of rats drowning in a water-filled beaker. This model is based on Seligman's "learned helplessness" model of human depression. It is, however, impossible to determine why bupropion-treated rats swim longer. Perhaps they are less depressed. Perhaps they are relieved of a "panic attack" type syndrome. Perhaps they are affected physiologically, for example, by muscle excitation or increased respiratory drive.

Even though animal modelers attribute bupropion's discovery to the animal models of depression, this is not valid for two reasons. First, the animal models are of doubtful relevance to human depression. Second, the animal tests did not indicate strongly that bupropion would prove an effective antidepressant. The bupropion story is typical: A clinical hypothesis (i.e., amphetamine's known mood-altering effect) prompted the animal modelers' work. In conclusion, animal experiments cannot reliably predict human reactions, just as they cannot confirm or disprove human-derived data. Medical researchers, however, continue to point to laboratory results *when those results appear to support their hypotheses.*

Critique of Current System of Psychoactive Drug Development

Currently, psychoactive drug development consists largely of screening analogues of known antidepressant or antipsychotic compounds with animal models or with *in vitro* receptor binding assays. While the value of receptor binding assays is now undergoing evaluation, the track record of animal models in psychopharmacologic drug screening is notoriously poor. S. Gershon notes that the results of psychopharmacologic efficacy experiments on animals have not significantly correlated with efficacy in patients.[25] Sitaram and Gershon have concluded:

> Two major points emerge from our readings; the surprisingly poor track record of most if not all animal models to date (a) in accurately predicting clinically effective antidepressants and (b) in generating new and conceptually liberating hypotheses of the pathophysiology of depression. These observations are highlighted by the fact that almost every significant advance in antidepressant drug treatment from the discovery of iproniazid and imipramine to the recently introduced "second generation" class of antidepressants has resulted either from astute clinical observations or serendipity; a far cry from a planned, predictive, screening test. In fact

> many second generation antidepressants such as iprindol, mianserin, trazodone and salbutamol should be classified as "false negatives" on the conventional drug screening models (i.e., ineffective during preclinical screening but clinically efficacious). Conversely, a series of compounds, predicted to be at least as effective as imipramine, were reported to be clinically ineffective (i.e., false positives).[26]

Given the low preclinical-clinical correlation, animal behavior tests appear to be a poor method for screening congeners of parent psychoactive compounds. Gershon notes that the second and third generation antidepressants are not clearly more effective than the parent compounds originally detected in human studies in the 1950s and 1960s. Gershon and co-authors comment, "One wonders about those compounds that might have been clinically useful but could not make it through these conventional tests. Whether the 'censorship' practiced by these animal models prevented us from developing novel antidepressants remains an unanswered question."[27]

In defiance of their own observations, Sitaram and Gershon go on to express confidence that improved animal models will show greater utility.[26] Animal models are unlikely to lead to the development of novel drugs for treating depression, schizophrenia, bipolar disorders, and other psychological disorders. It is impossible to determine the extent to which artificially induced psychological "disorders" in nonhuman animals resemble the psychiatric syndromes of human patients. Green and Costain have noted fundamental problems with the animal models: "We do not believe there is any totally satisfactory animal model of psychiatric disorder. Drugs cannot therefore be given to a 'pathological' brain to make it normal but rather to a 'normal' brain, thereby perhaps changing it to an 'abnormal' state. Changes that occur may thus be of a reflection of brain neurotransmitter systems attempting to minimize the changes being produced by the drug."[28] Animal models of human psychological disorders are inherently flawed -- at best, inaccurate; at worst, completely invalid.

The anomalous CNS side-effects of marketed drugs have inspired past psychopharmaceutical discoveries. Davis, reviewing the historical record, recognizes the importance of the clinical setting as a source of psychoactive drug discovery:

> Many of the psychotropic drugs were discovered by chance when they were administered for one indication and observed to be helpful for an entirely different condition. The history of the development of both the antidepressants and the antipsychotic drugs points up the fact that major scientific discoveries can evolve as a consequence of clinical investigation, rather than

deductions from basic animal research.[29]

Postmarketing Surveillance and Psychoactive Drug Discovery

Clinical pharmacologist L. Lasagna of Tuft University has written, "I agree that most of the prototype drugs in psychopharmacology were discovered by smart clinicians who saw things happen in humans that were not expected (chlorpromazine, imipramine, LSD, benzodiazepines)."[15] Given that the process of drug discovery for mental illness relies on identifying mood-altering side-effects, new classes of psychoactive compounds are unlikely to be discovered outside the clinical setting. The implications for research strategy are unambiguous: It is essential to systematically monitor marketed drugs' side-effects on the human CNS. In the U.S., postmarketing surveillance (PMS) is still in a rudimentary stage.

The potential of PMS as a means of drug discovery has not gone unrecognized. In 1980, in the Final Report of the Joint Commission on Prescription Drug Use, Melmon wrote:

> Another objective of PMS is to discover beneficial drug effects (anticipated or unanticipated) after a drug has been marketed. Although it is not possible to systematize serendipitous discoveries, it is desirable to approach the discovery of new indications for drugs more systematically. For example, careful follow-up of published reports of new effects of marketed drugs . . . or the monitoring of trends in medical events (e.g., cardiovascular deaths) in our population may provide useful clues about unanticipated beneficial effects of drugs. This objective is by no means a trivial one, as many additional beneficial effects of drugs have been discovered after the drugs have been approved for marketing. Such discovery is not only beneficial for populations having a disease treatable by the new use of an approved drug, but also represents an improvement in safety and economy in drug development, since many new uses may reduce the cost of development and simultaneously prevent unnecessary exposure of subjects to potentially toxic and/or ineffective experimental drugs.[30]

McIlwain contends that most drugs affect the human CNS in some way.[1] Consequently, the potential of PMS to uncover novel psychiatric medications appears to be bright. Indeed, the clinic continues to produce promising psychoactive drugs. In 1990, Greenberg noted that a schizophrenic patient responded dramatically to famotidine, a histamine H_2 receptor antagonist that the patient was receiving as treatment for peptic ulcer disease.[31]

Robinson and Kurtz, too, have noted the potential of PMS to uncover drugs with which to treat brain disorders:

> Perhaps a look into the past can give a glimpse of the future. In this regard, the potential of serendipity cannot be overlooked when evaluating treatment strategies. Throughout the history of medicine, there are examples of significant advances coming about as a result of careful clinical monitoring of a drug that was supposed to do something else but had an effect in an unpredicted direction. Iproniazid [which caused euphoria] in tuberculosis patients leading to the new class of [antidepressant] monoamine oxidase inhibitors is an outstanding example, as are the tricyclic antidepressants originally developed as antipsychotics.[32]

In conclusion, post-marketing surveillance is potentially the most efficient and reliable strategy for discovering new psychopharmaceutical agents.

Acknowledgement: I would like to thank the Ahimsa Foundation, whose support made this project possible.

References

1. McIlwain M: *Chemotherapy and the Central Nervous System*. Boston, Little Brown & Co, 1959.
2. Swazey J: *Chlorpromazine in Psychiatry: A Study in Therapeutic Innovation*. Cambridge, MIT Press, 1974.
3. Campion FD: *The AMA and U.S. Health Policy since 1940*. Chicago, Chicago Review Press, 1984.
4. Reines BP: On the locus of medical discovery. *The Journal of Medicine and Philosophy,*in press.
5. Caldwell A: *Origins of Psychopharmacology: From CPZ to LSD*. Sprinfield, Charles C Thomas, 1970.
6. Anon: Serendipity in discovery of benzodiazepines. *Psychiatric Times*, September, 1987.
7. Kuhn R: Über die behandlung depressiver zustande mit einemiminodibenzylderivat (G22355). *Schweiz Med Wochenschn* 1957;87:1135-1140.
8. Sulser F, Mishra R: The discovery of tricyclic antidepressants and their mode of action, in Parnham MJ, Bruinvels J (eds): *Discoveries in Pharmacology: Volume 1, Psycho- and Neuro-pharmacology*. New York, Elsevier, 1983.
9. Haefely W: Alleviation of anxiety -- the benzodiazepine saga, in Parnham MJ, Bruinvels J (eds): *Discoveries in Pharmacology: Volume 1, Psycho- and Neuro-pharmacology*. New York, Elsevier, 1983.
10. Lehman H, Kline NS: Clinical discoveries with antidepressant drugs, in Parnham MJ, Bruinvels J (eds): *Discoveries in Pharmacology: Volume 1, Psycho- and Neuro-pharmacology*. New York, Elsevier, 1983.
11. Pincus HA, Fine T, Pardes H, Goodwin FK: The animal rights movement: A research perspective. *Am J Psychiat* 1986;143:1585-1586.
12. Goodwin F: We can't sacrifice people for the sake of animal life. *Newsday*, May 21,

1989.
13. Levine J, Schield B, Bouthilet L (eds): *Establishing the Efficacy of Psychotropic Agents.* PHS Pub No 2138, 1971.
14. Kline NS: Lithium: The history of its use in psychiatry. *Modern Problems in Pharmacopsychiatry* 1969;3:75-92.
15. Lasagna L: Personal communication, 1989.
16. Cade J: Lithium salts for the treatment of psychotic excitement. *Med J Austr* 1949;36:349-351.
17. Jefferson JW, Greist JH, Ackerman DL, Carroll JA: *Lithium Encyclopedia for Clinical Practice,* Second Edition. Washington, DC, American Psychiatric Press, 1987.
18. Johnson FN: *The History of Lithium Therapy.* London, Macmillan, 1984.
19. Cooper BR, Howard JL, Soroko FE: Animal models used in prediction of antidepressant effects in man. *J Clin Psychiat* 1983;44(5, sec 2):63-66.
20. Mehta NB: The chemistry of bupropion. *J Clin Psychiat* 1983;44(5 sec 2):56-59.
21. NDA 18-644, Burroughs-Wellcome Co, Dec 30, 1985, p 6.
22. Weintraub M, Evans P: Bupropion: A chemically and pharmacologically unique antidepressant. *Hosp Formul* 1989;24:254-259.
23. Mason AA, Granacher RP: *Clinical Handbook of Antipsychotic Drug Therapy.* New York, Brunner/Mazel, 1980.
24. Hollister LE: *Clinical Pharmacology of Psychotherapeutic Drugs*, Second Edition. New York, Churchill Livingstone, 1983.
25. Gershon S: Predictiveness in psychopharmacology: Preclinical-clinical correlations, in Wittenborn J (ed): *Psychopharmacology and the Individual Patient.* New York, Raven Press, 1970, pp 9-31.
26. Sitaram N, Gershon S: From animal models to clinical testing -- promises and pitfalls. *Prog Neuro-Psychopharmacol & Biol Psychiat* 1983;7:227-228.
27. Kelwala S, Stanley M, Gershon S: History of antidepressants: Successes and failures. *J Clin Psychiat* 1983;44(5, sec 2):40-48.
28. Green AR, Costain DW: *Pharmacology and Biochemistry of Psychiatric Disorders.* New York, John Wiley & Sons, 1981.
29. Davis JM: Antipsychotic drugs, in Kaplan HI, Sadock BJ (eds): *Comprehensive Textbook of Psychiatry,* Fourth Edition. Baltimore, Williams & Wilkins, 1985.
30. Melmon K: Testimony before the Subcommittee of Health and Scientific Research, Committee on Labor and Human Resources, US Senate. Washington, US Gov Printing Office, 1980.
32. Robinson DS, Kurtz NM: A scientific and pharmacological industry perspective, in Crook T, Bartus R, Ferris S, Gershon S (eds): *Treatment Strategies for Alzheimer's Disease.* New York, Mark Powley, 1986.
31. Gelengerg AJ: Famotidine for schizophrenia? *Biological Therapies in Psychiatry Newsletter* 1990;13(11).

Spheroid Cultures for Cancer Research and Treatment

Ron Allison, M.D.

Introduction

Spheroid models are sphere-shaped cell colonies that permit growth and function studies of diverse normal and malignant tissues. Spheroid growth mimics the growth of naturally occurring human tumors. In both, cells in contact with nutrients grow quickly while the kinetics and activity of cells further inward depend on diffusion.

Sophisticated microtechniques permit analysis of whole spheroids, spheroid subpopulations within the colony, or even individual cells. Manipulations of the spheroid environment have provided insights into tumor physiology, and research with therapeutic agents, such as radiation, offers hope for improved cancer treatment.

History

Since the late 1950s, multicellular aggregates of malignant cells have been analyzed for proliferation, differentiation, invasion potential, and structural similarity to human tumors on a large scale.[1] However, it was not until the early 1970s that Sutherland and coworkers systematically investigated the response of tumor cell aggregates to antineoplastic therapy. Because the cell lines formed nearly perfect sphere-shaped aggregates, they were called "spheroids."[2]

Spheroid Cultures

A wide range of normal and malignant cell types can be grown as spheroids. Embryonic, fetal, postnatal, and adult cells from virtually all organ systems, including the central nervous system, may be maintained in culture for several weeks. Recently, cells that would not form spheroids have been induced to do so by co-culturing with spheroid-forming non-clonogenic feeder cells.[3]

Histologic examination of these spheroids reveal striking similarities between their structure and that of naturally occurring human tumors. Furthermore, the response of culture spheroids to cancer therapy is so similar to the response obtained in humans that many investigators consider spheroids useful for studying cancer cells' basic biological properties.[4]

Spheroids may be used for studies of viability, clonogenicity, LD50, and metastatic potential under a variety of experimental conditions. In certain systems, spheroids can be mechanically or chemically "peeled like an onion" so that specific cell subpopulations can be isolated and studied.[5] Research on spheroids grown from a biopsy of a patient's tumor may one day allow individualized treatment that would increase the chance of a cure.

Common Characteristics of Spheroids and Tumors

Analysis of human tumors and their spheroid counterparts has revealed numerous structural, functional, and biological similarities.[6] Structurally, spheroids are virtually indistinguishable from samples taken from the original tumor. Functional analysis of spheroids reveals that their secretory and metabolic activity is similar to that of the tumors or organs from which the spheroids derive. For example, human colon carcinoma spheroids secrete measurable quantities of carcinoembryonic antigen, thyroid cell spheroids produce thyroid hormones, and hepatocyte spheroids can exhibit the same metabolic functions as liver tissues. These characteristics are not necessarily seen when the same cells are cultured as monolayers.[4]

Biologically, both spheroids and natural tumors are composed of heterogeneous cells. In naturally occurring tumors, cells close to blood vessels are well-supplied with oxygen and nutrients, and they actively proliferate and secrete various substances. Cells farther from the nutrient vessels are progressively more hypoxic and acidic, grow more slowly, and appear to be relatively resistant to antineoplastic therapy.

Spheroids share these characteristics. Cells close to the sphere surface, in contact with oxygen and with environmental nutrients, actively proliferate and secrete various substances. Further inward, cell viability depends on diffusion of nutrients in and waste out. Interestingly, the areas of hypoxia in spheroid cultures occur 200 microns from the sphere surface, and analysis of human tumor biopsies reveals areas of hypoxia 200 microns from nutrient vessels.

Because the spheroid environment can be controlled and manipulated, milieu effects on tumor cell viability can be carefully examined. Using microtechniques and automated cell sorting, each cell can be evaluated and the effects of varied growth factors, such as nutrients, hormones, and therapeutic interventions, can be systematically studied and analyzed. Using these techniques, certain areas of spheroids have been identified that contain chronically hypoxic cells resistant to all forms of therapy. These studies, as well as research with human tumors *in vivo*, support the belief that the chronically hypoxic cells are often responsible for cancer treatment failure.[5,7] Much research is being conducted in the area of therapeutic techniques to promote cancer cell oxygenation. For example, hypoxic cells produce specific proteins,[8] and manipulation of these proteins may influence cell viability and growth.

Cell-to-cell communication within tumors can also be studied using spheroids. In spheroids, as in naturally occurring tumors, numerous communication channels, including gap junctions, desmosomes, and electrical coupling, develop. Studies of these processes may provide insight into molecular mechanisms regulating cell proliferation and differentiation.

An exciting area of research involves co-culturing normal cells with malignant cells within a spheroid. Tumor invasion of the normal cell often occurs. This technique, called "confrontation," appears to be a valid method of evaluating invasion.[9] Modifications, including the use of human amnion as tissue with spheroid tumor aggregates as metastatic lesions, have proved valuable in the study of metastasis.[10]

Spheroids are also used to elucidate immune factors in tumor dynamics. Sutherland developed an *in vitro* system analyzing the response of tumor spheroids to diverse human lymphocytes.[11] He found that diminished clonogenicity follows certain tumor-lymphocyte reactions. Another area of active research involves evaluation and modification of synthetic antibodies for therapeutic effect.

Therapy

Therapeutic interventions using spheroids have received wide attention. Modalities include radiation, chemotherapy, hyperthermia, immunotherapy and combinations of these. For example, researchers have found that irradiated spheroids are more resistant than monolayers to cell death because hypoxic areas within spheroids are radioresistant. Since hypoxic areas in naturally occurring tumor may limit curability, modification or elimination of these cells is necessary. One promising approach utilizes agents that label the hypoxic fraction.[12] Also, radiation sensitizing agents have been developed using spheroids for screening and testing,[5] but clinical efficacy remains to be determined. Interestingly, spheroid analysis has shown that multiple-dose radiation regimens, similar to those used clinically, are able to minimize hypoxic cell populations and increase cancer cell kill.[5,7]

Analysis of the effects of chemotherapeutic agents has shown that certain drugs will not diffuse far enough into spheroids to achieve adequate cell kill. Testing modified drug structure on spheroids can lead to agents of improved effectiveness.[13]

Certain cells within spheroids may develop genetic resistance. Perhaps new and more effective agents can be developed once these cells are isolated and evaluated. Additionally, by tagging the chemotherapeutic agents, microanalysis can reveal which cell sub-populations are most affected by particular drugs. In this way, combinations of chemotherapeutic agents may be evaluated to optimize tumor kill. Finally, new antiproliferative agents may be screened and analyzed using spheroids, which offer a promising approach to drug discovery.[13]

Spheroids have already modified immunotherapy. Initially, anti-tumor antibodies were too large to penetrate effectively into spheroid tumors. This was also true of antibodies used against human tumors. The use of spheroids to study immune therapy has led to a new generation of cytotoxic antibodies with increased tumor penetration.[14] These are in the process of clinical trials.

Eventually, spheroids grown from a patient's tumor may be used to test the efficacy of a wide range of therapeutic options. This approach is not readily accomplished using monolayer cell cultures because monolayers lack the extensive cell-to-cell contact, the hypoxic cell populations, and the variable cell cycle times seen in both spheroids and naturally occurring human tumors.[15] Most importantly, monolayer cultures generally employ established, immortal cell lines rather than biopsy specimens from actual tumors of patients. Because monolayers select for immortal cells, they may not be representative of most cells within a tumor. Nevertheless, monolayer cell cultures retain some value in screening new therapeutics because they are fully automated and reliable and many different human cell lines are available for testing.[16]

Use of animal models to screen therapeutic regimens and individualize therapy is not practical. The clinician cannot withhold cancer therapy for the months required to grow tumor cells in animals and to test treatment modalities.[5] Additionally, it is virtually impossible to obtain from the patient the amount of tumor mass needed for transplantation into the many animals required to test the many individual and combination therapies available. Also, the costs of animals, manpower, and laboratory space would be prohibitive. Most importantly, these systems are unreliable. While the tumor cells are of human origin, the animal's immune response, metabolism, and toxic response to therapy all influence outcome. Even inbred animal strains can have variable tumor responses.[5,17]

Future Applications

Spheroids are an established model for biological and therapeutic studies of malignancy. They are reliable, reproducible, and economical.[5] As technology advances, the applications of spheroids will increase. High resolution MRI, MRS, and PET are already being used to evaluate tumor physiology within intact spheroids. Perhaps the greatest contribution of spheroids will come once the biopsies of cancer patients are grown as spheroids. These cultures may then serve to individualize and optimize the best therapies available. This approach is currently under evaluation by the Radiation Therapy Oncology Group, a consortium of leading clinical and experimental radiation oncologists.

References

1. Moscona A: The development *in vitro* of chimeric aggregates of dissociated embryonic chick and mouse cells. *Proc Natl Acad Sci* 1957;43:184-194.
2. Sutherland RM, McCredie JA, Inch WR: Growth of multicellular spheroids in tissue culture as a model of nodular carcinomas. *J Nat Canc Inst* 1971;46:113-120.
3. Djordjevic B, Lange C: Clonogenicity of mammalian cells in hybrid spheroids: A new assay method. *Radiat Environ Biophys* 1990;29:31-46.
4. Mueller-Klieser W: Multicellular spheroids. *J Canc Res Clin Onc* 1987;113:101-22.
5. Hall EJ: *Radiobiology for the radiologist.* Philadelphia, Lippincott, 1988.
6. Nederman T, Norling B, Glemelius B, Carlsson J, Bruntz U: Demonstration of an extracellular matrix in multicellular spheroids. *Cancer Res* 1984;44:3090-3097.
7. Sutherland RM: Cell-environment interaction in tumor microregions: The multicell spheroid model. *Science* 1988;240;177-184.
8. Freyer JP, Sutherland RM: Regulation of growth saturation in the development of necrosis in spheroids. *Cancer Res* 1986;46:3504.
9. Schleich A: The confrontation of normal and malignant cells *in vitro*, in Garattino S (ed): *Chemotherapy of Cancer Dissemination with Metastasis*. New York, Raven Press, 1973, pp 51-58.
10. Marcel MM: The use of culture to study invasion *in vitro*, in Liotta LA, Hart IR (eds): *Tumor Invasion and Metastases.* The Hague, Martinus Nijhoff, 1982, pp 207-230.
11. Sutherland RM, MacDonald HR, Howell RL: Multicellular spheroids: A new model target for *in vitro* studies of immunity. *J Nat Canc Inst* 1977;58:1849-1853.
12. Franko AJ: Hypoxic fraction with binding of misonidazole in multicellular tumor spheroids. *Radiation Tes* 1985;103:89-97.
13. Mederman T: Growth of tumor cells as spheroids and antitumor drug evaluations, in Dendy PP, Hall BT (eds): *Human Tumor Drug Testing In Vitro.* London, Academic Press,

1983, pp 147-161.
14. Sutherland RM, Buchegger F, Shreyer M, Vacca A, Mach J-P:Penetration and Binding of radiolabeled anti-carcinoembryonic antigen monoclonal antibodies and their antigen binding fragments in human colon multicellular tumor spheroids. *Cancer Res* 1987;47:1627-1633.
15. Sutherland R, Durand R: Radiation response in multicell spheroids. *Current Topics Radiation Res* 1976;11:87-139.
16. Boyd M: Status of the NCI preclinical antitumor drug discovery screen. *PPO Updates of Cancer* 1989;Oct(10).
17. Kallman R: *Rodent Tumors in Experimental Cancer Therapy.* New York, Pergamon, 1987.

Review of Scoliosis Research at the University of Michigan

Joel D. Mack, M.D. and Robert A. Greenberg, M.D.

Scoliosis is a spine curvature that can considerably disable humans. About 75-80% of scoliosis cases are idiopathic; the rest are caused by musculoskeletal abnormalities, neuromuscular diseases, trauma, nerve root compression, spinal cord tumors, and other conditions.[1] The etiology of idiopathic scoliosis is unknown; a better understanding of the causes of scoliosis may improve scoliosis management. However, it is difficult, if not impossible, for animal models to provide clinically relevant insights into human idiopathic scoliosis: artificial induction of scoliosis in animals does not parallel spontaneous human scoliosis, and the erect human has fundamentally different forces on the spine than four-legged animals. Having reviewed a research grant proposal submitted by J.A. Ashton Miller[2] to study spinal muscle functions in a canine model of scoliosis, we conclude that there are severe methodological flaws.

Ashton Miller claims three general points of significance for this study. First, he writes, "This proposal is aimed at improving our understanding of the mechanisms of curve progression in scoliosis."[2] While this issue has therapeutic and prognostic importance, the value of these dog studies is dubious. Ashton Miller plans to induce experimental scoliosis in dogs by external forces. It is unlikely that this artificial protocol reproduces the situation in human scoliosis. Also, the rate of scoliosis formation in the animal model differs dramatically from that in humans. Ashton Miller notes:

> In man, the *average* curve progression rate seldom exceeds 10 degrees per year. Of course, it would have been best to study similar rates in dog [sic]. However, firstly we are not assured that trends in the muscular response to such slow rates can reliably be detected given the noise in myoelectric estimates of muscle contraction intensity and secondly, the study of an adequate number of animals to achieve statistical significance over 12 months or longer is prohibitively expensive.[2]

Range of curve progression will vary between 10 degrees per hour to 5 degrees per week, all of which greatly exceed normal curve progression in humans. This raises the possibility that he will be studying artifactual consequences of rapid scoliosis induction, rather than the real progression of scoliosis.

A second area of significance, according to Ashton Miller, is that "There are no longitudinal studies of paravertebral muscle response to the presence of scoliosis."[2] He continues, "Usually, attention has been focused exclusively on the convex and concave sides of the curve apex, rather than at multiple levels as in the present proposal."[2] Myoelectric studies have been done on human scoliotic patients, and it is possible that Ashton Miller's electromyographic data could be gathered from human clinical subjects. Indeed, Ashton Miller proposes to perform simultaneous human clinical studies in an effort to validate the animal model. If it were possible to obtain the desired information safely and ethically with human patients, then the animal studies would be superfluous. Ashton Miller, recognizing the limitations of animal models, writes, "Extrapolation of the results from dogs to the human case is fraught with uncertainties."[2] Consequently, an animal model appears to be inappropriate.

Ashton Miller concludes:

> The significance of the animal experiments is that we will, for the first time, study the spatial and temporal response of the intact musculoskeletal system to ramp and step changes in the magnitude of an experimentally-induced scoliosis. This may be done in animal experiments at a level of detail not normally possible in the clinical setting. . . . The significance of this proposal is the recognition of the importance of understanding the muscular response to a scoliosis.[2]

Although Ashton Miller contends that he will obtain useful data, the relevance of this animal model is doubtful. Ashton Miller appears to misunderstand the nature of scoliosis. He writes, "Scoliosis, or a lateral curvature of the spine, occurs in about 3% of adolescents."[2] This is inaccurate. In fact, scoliosis generally has a rotational component,[3,4] which may be the more important component of the deformity. Roaf has summarized:

> There are two types of scoliosis, which occur independently of etiology. The first is an uncommon type in which lateral flexion is the dominant element. The curve usually remains relatively mobile, is fairly easily corrected, has less tendency to relapse after fusion, and presents minimal rib deformity; basically it is an exaggeration of a normal movement.
>
> The other type of curve, in which rotation is the main feature, tends to be progressive; it soon becomes rigid and resistant to correction, and tends to relapse after fusion for two reasons. Firstly, there is an internal torsion

> and asymmetry of the vertebrae themselves which are largely confined to the neural arch. . . . Secondly, in consequence of the rotation, six secondary deforming factors come into action which inevitably tend to increase the deformity.[4]

Thus, lateral deformity of the spine rarely causes severe clinical problems, but the more common variety of scoliosis, which has a rotation component, often causes disabilities. Ashton Miller's model, at best, addresses the less common type of scoliosis.

A further problem with this animal model is that the dog's quadruped structure results in markedly different forces on the spine than occurs in the biped human. Ashton Miller writes:

> Although dog [sic] as a quadruped is a less-than-ideal model for studying the musculoskeletal response of the bipedal spine, there are some redeeming features that make it reasonable to start with. In upright man the primary loading of the spine is axial compression arising from trunk extensor response to the forward flexion moment due to trunk weight. Any lateral movements arising from the body weight, inertia or muscle action must be equilibrated by muscles lateral to the spine. In dog, the primary loading is compression due to trunk flexor response to the extension moment created by bodyweight. Lateral movements arising from inertial effects or muscle action must be equilibrated by muscles lateral to the spine. So, although the basic spine compression loading may arise for different reasons in the two situations, the lateral movements which can arise in scoliosis must be equilibrated in a similar manner.[1]

Although Ashton Miller dismisses the musculoskeletal differences between dogs and humans, erect posture has important implications for human scoliosis. Erect posture puts gravitational force on the spine, which increases the curvature. X-ray evaluation of scoliosis patients always includes erect views, in order to assess the contribution of the gravitational forces to the scoliosis.[3]

In any case, experimental artifact may invalidate the research results. The "spine compression devices" used to induce scoliosis will, like all foreign bodies, induce scarring of the surrounding tissues, including the muscles. This will likely affect those muscles' functioning. This renders the research results uninterpretable.

Ashton Miller finishes his "Significance" section with the observation, "Finally, but not least, the success of this proposal would launch the investigator on an independent research career in the area of spine biomechanics." Career advancement hardly seems a proper reason for either conducting such research or receiving funds to do so. The history of artificially induced scoliosis in a dog differs markedly from the natural history of human scoliosis. Any data obtained by Ashton Miller will be of questionable relevance to humans.

This project, funded by the Public Health Service, represents an inappropriate use of research dollars.

References

1. Edmonson AS: Scoliosis, in Crenshaw AH (ed): *Campbell's Operative Orthopedics, Seventh Edition*. St Louis, CV Mosby, 1987.
2. Ashton Miller JA: Muscle activity in congenital and experimental scoliosis. PHS Grant application 85-716-J1, submitted 10/22/84 for funding from 7/1/85 to 6/30/88.
3. Winter RB: The spine, in Lovell WW, Winter RB (eds): *Pediatric Orthopedics*. Philadelphia, JB Lippincott, 1978, pp 573-584.
4. Roaf R: Rotation movements of the spine with special reference to scoliosis. *J Bone Joint Surg* 1958;40B:312-332.

Debunking Myths in Nursing Theory and Research*

Peggy L. Chinn, R.N., Ph.D., F.A.A.N.

Abstract

This article examines myths that persist in the traditional male-defined scientific enterprise. Science *per se* is not rejected, but specific ways of confronting the myths are explored. The methods for debunking the myths derive from the concept of future search, wherein health and the values of nursing for the future direct the discovery of knowledge. The alternatives include a more ethical and responsible use of the methods of science as well as specific alternatives to science derived from Carper's[1] patterns of knowing in nursing.

The nursing literature has reflected growing recognition of the limitations of the scientific method in addressing problems in nursing.[2-7] Taken together, the literature leaves the impression that we should perhaps forsake the scientific method; alternatives for acquiring knowledge in nursing are not adequately described, and the alternatives that are suggested are not clearly alternatives to the traditional scientific method.

Most critiques of the scientific method fail to recognize that traditional science is based on a male world view and that the myths sustained by this partial world view have perpetuated erroneous knowledge about the world. The purposes of this article are (a) to present an analysis of myths of science that arise from the partial male world view, (b) to propose methods for debunking these myths to attain a more whole science consistent with the essence of nursing, and (c) to propose alternative approaches to science where an alternative is indicated.

Myths

The concept of "myth" carries many meanings. Two dictionary definitions focus attention on the meanings that are relevant to the focus of this article: "a traditional story of ostensibly historical events that serves to unfold part of the world view of a people, or explain a practice, belief, or natural phenomenon" and "an ill-founded belief held uncritically, especially by an interested

* This essay, in modified form, is reprinted by permission of *Image: The Journal of Nursing Scholarship.*

group."[8]

Myths remain a powerful force in the creation of sociocultural patterns, and science and scientists are equally subject to their influence. Myths are not entirely false and in fact contain an element of reality. This is why they are so seductive and difficult to recognize. Since myths are based on a particular world view, they function actually to shape and create reality. Until we examine myths critically, we are not able to sort out what is ill-founded from that which is well-founded, or whose interest are served.

Traditional science has created beliefs about reality that are taken to be "true." Current scientific enterprise, however, rests on a white, upper-class male view of the world.[9] This view is not necessarily wrong or bad, but it is not universal. Regardless of the actual origins of the prevailing world view or whether it arose from the maleness *per se*, it focuses on attributes and phenomena traditionally considered "male": power, control, instrumentation, technology, competition, rationality, logic, objectivity, hard data. Not only does this view rest on the superiority of male-assigned traits, but it also disdains concepts that are consistent with that which is assigned as being "feminine": soft data, subjectivity, feeling, emotion, intuition, and so forth. This arbitrary value assignment clearly does not serve the interests of nursing or the best interest of humanity. Spender discussed the myth of the superiority of that which is masculine in language:

> The myth was made a long time ago and for centuries it has been fostered by women and men so that now it is deeply embedded in virtually every aspect of our existence. It is a myth which may be attacked but one which is not easy to eradicate, for all myths still have a hold over us long after they have been intellectually repudiated, and this one, which is fundamental to our social order, is particularly pervasive and particularly hard to dislodge. The fabric of our social organization has been woven to support and substantiate it and nothing less than a restructuring of our beliefs and values is necessary, if it is to be laid to rest.[10]

Future Search

Just as language is a powerful tool for conveying the prevailing world view, an examination of new meanings for language can be used to create a shift. The word "research" is a useful starting point. The activities that happen under the name of research are often literally re-searching what has been done over and over again. Usually the hypotheses shift from project to project, but there is seldom any creativity in the conceptualizations or methods used primarily because credibility depends on doing the same thing (or close to it) in the same way. What this does is perpetuate the *status quo* -- a past-oriented perspective.

Heide[11] proposes that we shift our focus to future search. Future search requires that we envision the world as it could be, or as we want it to be -- a healthy, productive, peaceful, enduring, nurturing environment and society. Once we have this vision, we can begin to discover knowledge that is required to create this world. As nursing scholars, we can end the perpetuation of a *status quo* that values illness more than health; we can enact what we know in our practice by focusing our scholarly energies in the direction of health for all. In short, we can be change agents.[12]

Future-search methods that serve to debunk myths in nursing science rests on the following assumptions:

* Nursing's world view is both reasonable and valuable. This world view focuses on health, life, human interaction, and environmental integrity. Further, nursing has incorporated values traditionally deemed "feminine" -- values in conflict with much of current scientific enterprise.
* The traditional scientific method is useful for some questions but not for all questions.
* In conceptualizing methods of generating knowledge, it is not useful to think in terms of dichotomies of "scientific" and "nonscientific." Other analogous concepts include "the received view" vs. the "non-received view"[7] and "paradigm I logic" vs. "paradigm II logic."[13] These dichotomies imply that science remains the standard for judging all methods. Future search views traditional science as one method, but not the standard for judging all methods.
* The appeal in the literature for alternative methods and logical systems is valid, and the types of knowledge that are required in nursing have been described.[1] However, the methods are yet to be created, described, or demonstrated to be useful.

The Myths of Re-Search

There are several ways to approach a movement toward future search. The movement begins with debunking myths of the scientific enterprise. In considering the myths, I am not suggesting that we eliminate the concepts entirely; I am suggesting that we debunk these ideas as sacred truths, examine the dimensions of these ideas that are partial or false, and move in a direction of wholeness consistent with our world view.

Myth #1: The Myth of the Ultimate Truth

The myth of the ultimate truth leads us to think that science represents some absolute reality. Scientific theory is supposed to represent reality, and reality is supposed to be truth. Truth, as it is conceptualized in the traditional scientific enterprise, is represented in the assumptions of theories and research. For the most part, the assumptions are rarely recognized much less questioned. By subscribing to the assumptions as "truth," we seek data that conform to our view and ignore contrary evidence that does not support the underlying assumption of what is true. We ignore as being idiosyncratic (insignificant) data that do not conform to our preconceived beliefs.

The method for debunking this myth is to identify existing assumptions. Once existing assumptions are identified, contrary evidence will not be automatically dismissed, but will simply be incorporated into an enlarged viewpoint.

The work of Gilligan[14] demonstrates the importance of questioning underlying "truths" and unstated assumptions. Gilligan studied with Kohlberg and learned his theory of moral development. Later, she realized there was important information that had not been disclosed in final reports of the research or integrated into the theory. Kohlberg's theory is based on all-male research. When the theory and tools derived from it were used with women, women were found not to achieve development beyond the third state of a 10-stage process and were assumed to be inferior to men.[14] Gilligan reexamined the theory and questioned the assumption that failing to be "10" represents an inferiority. Using methods of traditional science, she demonstrated contrary evidence required to debunk the myth of the universality of Kohlberg's theory, revealing that women are not inferior; the theory is inferior. In a very fundamental way, Kohlberg's theory does not withstand the test of universality, as Kohlberg has claimed. In the process of discovering contrary evidence, Gilligan also contributed knowledge that has begun to change how women are viewed -- a hallmark of the future search enterprise.[15]

Myth #2: The Myth of Objectivity

Traditional science prides itself on being "value-free" and therefore objective and not subjective. Intellectually, some traditional scientists recognize that no science is value-free; nor is it free from subjective influence. However, it is not the value laden bias of the scientific enterprise that is the problem; it is the continuing failure to acknowledge and take seriously the nature of the values and subjective interpretations that are imposed on the so-called "objective" ideas, methods, and designs.

One of the dictionary meanings of "objective" is particularly enlightening: "methods that eliminate the subjective by limiting choices to fixed alternatives requiring a minimum of creative interpretation (e.g., tests of personality)."[8] Of course, the dictionary does not ask, "Who determined the alternatives? What values influenced their choice of the 'fixed alternatives?' Who decided that it was desirable to eliminate the 'subjective' and 'creative' in the testing of personality?"

The most insidious technique used to perpetrate the myth of objectivity is the erasure, abdication, and obfuscation of responsibility, thereby obscuring the subjective influence. The scientific literature, including that of nursing, is abundant with such phrases as "research results show" (What research? What kind of research? By whom?), and "it is generally known that" (By whom?). This is a tradition that works well to obscure responsibility and should be a major ethical concern for all scientists of our day. It is both an individual and a collective problem.

The method for debunking the myth of objectivity is to name the responsible agent, and to demystify the assumptions, the motives, the values, and the processes that were used to arrive at the definition of what is purported to be objective. We have a wonderful example in our own history of a nursing scholar who recognized this problem and took a strong stand opposing it. Writing in the *American Journal of Nursing* in 1915, Lavinia Dock stated:

> As a result of the European war, there are reappearances of ailments that were practically non-existent. Gaseous gangrene, never seen in surgery now-a-days, has come again. . . . When we know how surely and certainly these diseases are caused by men's own acts and deeds, does it not seem as if we should say, "Man's actions have produced gas-gangrene and typhus;" instead of the flabby statement, "Typhus is prevalent; gas-gangrene is developing." Seeing such ruthless and dastardly energies at work, does one not understand Florence Nightingale's impatient contempt for the germ theory, and comprehend her insistence that it was the things people did that caused disease?[16]

Exposing responsibility exposes underlying assumptions and myths and creates a new view of reality. For example, Florence Nightingale experienced the horrors of war and the destruction of human life and health; she refused to accept that the unsanitary conditions that she witnessed were "natural."

Her personal and subjective response to these conditions created an awareness of reality that was not generally accessible to other scholars of her day. Margaret Sanger grieved for the waste of human life and human potential that was created by the uncontrolled frequency of pregnancy, and she refused to assume that this condition was "natural." Her subjective, self-acknowledged response created the motive to seek the knowledge that would create health.

Myth #3: The Myth of the Perfect Method

The myth of the perfect method results in compulsive orderliness, repetition, and a fixation on minute details. It encourages us toward mental laziness in envisioning alternative methods, alternative approaches, and alternative assumptions. We re-search and re-search to the point that we know more and more about less and less, failing to recognize the relevance or irrelevance of what we are studying. The perfect method, by definition, leads us on a path of examining small segments and parts of reality apart from the whole and is based on the assumption that a segmented analysis of the parts will yield knowledge of the whole.

The method for debunking this myth begins with the recognition that there is no one perfect method and that various methods must be used in relation to each question that is asked. Most important, this shift requires valuing alternative methods in a fundamental way. It requires refusing to apologize for what is presumed to be inadequate when contrasted with the "perfect method." It also requires that we cease to view alternative methods as merely stepping stones to the "perfect method" or entirely different approaches (such as those I will describe in the following section), are to be used and developed for their own worth and value.

Nursing is faced with what might be called an imperative to debunk this myth arising from the nature of the work we do, what we have identified as important, and how we view our goals. In conceptualizing health, the client, the environment, and the nurse-client interactions, a clear holistic view has emerged. If we remain committed to this foundational view, then the traditional method, which requires studying parts or segments of things or people, is simply not adequate.[4] A segmented, partial approach might serve to enlighten or might serve some limited pragmatic purpose; it might be preferable to adapt the traditional methods to complex problems rather than to do nothing; however, as new methods emerge, they must be judged on their own merits, not against the false "standard" of the perfect method.

Myth #4: The Myth of Scientific Supremacy

The myth of scientific supremacy focuses on the religious-like quality of traditional science as the means for delineating truth, knowledge, and reality -- and as an end in and of itself. A critical component of this myth is the rejection of any other possibility for creating knowledge. Traditional science, which is based on the notion of empirical validation, is thought to result in true knowledge; all other forms of knowledge are judged as being merely speculation, opinion, or not what can be conceptualized as knowledge. If this myth did not have a strong hold on us, we would long ago have begun serious work to develop other ways of knowing.

Traditional science has served well to debunk myths perpetuated by the ancient philosophies and religions, and it is undoubtedly an effective way to obtain knowledge. However, science as the supreme end in and of itself has produced knowledge that has not turned out to be in the best human interest; indeed it has been used to create planet-wide contamination and has brought us to the brink of world-wide destruction.

The method for debunking the myth of scientific supremacy is to insist on the integration of the different patterns of knowing. The patterns of knowing described by Carper[1] derive from the nursing literature and serve well as a basis for envisioning that which is possible. Any one pattern of knowing used in isolation of the others is an incomplete, partial form of knowing. All patterns must be integrated to create what I would call Knowledge. Each pattern requires its own process of discovery and its own method for determining what is credible, as distinguished from isolated fantasy:

* Empirical knowledge is determined to be credible using empirical validation. This process requires verification -- agreement that what is observed by one person in one situation is replicable in other instances by other observers. The evidence used to judge credibility is what we know as reliability and validity.
* Ethical knowledge is determined to be credible by the method of justification. The philosophic and logical premises surrounding an ethical dilemma are stated explicitly, and from these are derived logical evidence that justifies a decision, or a conclusion. Other observers do not have to agree with the decision, but the decision, the evidence that produces the decision, and the logic used must be judged to be responsible and just.
* Esthetics is judged to be credible through the method of criticism.

Criticism as used in the arts is directed toward knowing, making explicit, exposing the meaning of the creative process/product. Consensus, or agreement among observers, related to meaning is not required but, for the criticism to function as a method for revealing credible esthetic meaning, consistency must exist between the expressions of the esthetic process and the criticism of it.

* Personal knowledge is determined to be credible through introspection. Introspection makes it possible to integrate and actualize that which is experienced in relation to others and the self. As introspection occurs, the authenticity of the self is revealed, and personal knowledge is actualized.

Myth #5: The Myth of Empirical Evidence

The myth of empirical evidence is the belief that "what is" is observable through sensory experience, and whatever is not observable through sensory experience does not exist. Furthermore, whatever is observable is measurable; it is quantifiable. The fundamental usefulness of empirical validation of phenomena is not to be rejected, but the myth represents a good idea gone wild. The myth extends the value of empirical validation of phenomena to encompass the belief that, if something cannot be empirically validated, it does not exist or is not worth pursuing. Further, the myth sustains the tendency to proclaim that something either is or is not empirically accessible when in reality phenomena are relatively accessible to empirical knowing. Science has stimulated ideas that give rise to possibilities for empirical validation long before empirical validation is possible; we call this the discovery of instrumentation, or methods for empirical observations. As we have moved into areas of knowledge that are relatively inaccessible, we create methods that are increasingly indirect in relations to the phenomena, still naming the indirect measure "empirical evidence" to justify the scientific nature of our enterprise. Once this is done, we call the phenomenon empirically validated: it exists.

As we leap through these mental exercises, we fail to seriously confront the artifacts that are created in the process of "empirical validation." I am not arguing that highly abstract phenomena (e.g., health or motive) cannot and should not be empirically validated; nor do I reject scholarly work in this direction; but I reject the assumption that empirical tools or observations are adequate to create comprehensive knowledge of these phenomena. I also question the assumption that empirical evidence itself will produce accurate knowledge.

The method for confronting the myth of empirical evidence is to recognize the limitations of empirical evidence in relation to developing knowledge and to value other ways of knowing related to the phenomena that we are exploring. As we recognize the limitations of empirical evidence, we can begin to untangle distortions that are created by artifacts of empirical validation. The untangling process will include improvements in our approaches to obtain empirical evidence as well as open possibilities for knowledge that do not derive from empirical evidence. I submit that our body of knowledge of a phenomenon such as "motive" in relation to health will ultimately require strong, sound empirical evidence free of artifacts. But the complex keys to understanding this and other phenomena do not reside solely with the scope of empirical validation. The key to understanding these complex phenomena requires integration of the methods of justification, criticism, and introspection.

Myth #6: The Myth of Higher Authority

The myth of higher authority governs the scientific enterprise in a number of ways. It perpetuates ethical, empirical, and moral dishonesty. Most scholarly work begins with a review of "authoritative" literature, and we use the authority of existing literature to justify everything we do. The halo effect that an idea or a belief acquires by being published is a remarkable transition that I can only perceive as being magic.

The very fact of being engaged in the academic/scientific enterprise confers a socially sanctioned aura of authority. We are in a position to give or withhold information at will; to use, coerce, and manipulate people with little if any challenge to our authority. Even the language we use in research communicates authority -- *control, manipulation* (of variables, conditions, numbers, people), *inference, standardization, operationalization, subjects, instruments*.

Being a scientist also confers the authority to assign value judgments and worth to phenomena, ideas, or things. The act of measuring produces dichotomous thinking, or hierarchical assignment of value. We speak of high and low, we rank order things and assign values to those things without questioning the meaning of the valuing or the contextual possibilities that might exist or be created by our valuing. This myth has made it possible for male scientists to assign the value of "the norm" to maleness. Simply assigning a value does not make a thing true or right, but assigning a value of "ten" creates the illusion of truth or rightness.

The method for debunking the myth of higher authority is to place ourselves in the position of the grass-roots people with whom we work, or for whom our knowledge might have the most direct effect. In essence, this strategy is one of ethical justification, esthetic criticism, and personal introspection. We must discard the myth that the scientific enterprise is by definition a higher authority and that the scientist by definition has rights or authorities that are different from those of any other individual. Once we make this shift in our thinking, we can examine how well our approaches, our methods, and our conclusions are consistent with experiential reality.

Myth #7: The Myth of Significance

The myth of significance is most clearly recognized by examining the statistical concept of significance. When we are told that something is "significant" at the .01 level of probability, it assumes a halo effect of significance far beyond the strictly technical and statistical meaning of the term. The statistician and the researcher (hopefully) know the limitations and restrictive meaning of the term "significance" in a statistical sense. However, scientists rarely adhere to the strict statistical meaning in interpreting their results. As long as the results reach statistical significance, the findings have meaning. If the results do not reach statistical significance, the findings must be explained and have little meaning. The "significance" of the results of studies is used to imply not the statistical concept but the more common language understanding of the term: that it is important. Rarely does anyone ask, "Significant for what? For whom? In what context?" We seldom ask for what purpose, or in whose interest, a scientific enterprise has been undertaken. These factors are critical in determining how much importance we attach to the results of our research -- those that are statistically significant as well as those that are not.

The method for debunking the myth of significance is to apply the test of importance in relation to future search purposes and goals, regardless of the statistical findings. By shifting our attention to the importance of the research, we can detect ways in which the research may or may not contribute to knowledge that can create the kind of world in which we wish to live and work.

We will discover many subtle ways in which our scientific enterprise limits the universality of the theories and the generalizability of the research. A statistically significant study that is based on white, male, middle-class values, that draws on a white, male, middle-class population (as in much nursing research), probably has little or no meaning, much less importance, for the majority of people in this world who are not white, middle-class, or male.

Why Debunk Myths?

In conclusion, I want to acknowledge that there are pitfalls in taking a skeptical view of the *status quo*, even though scientists are by definition supposed to be skeptical. My interpretations of the myths of the scientific enterprise are deliberately severe to stimulate awareness of the actual behavioral practices of many scientists and the flaws in that which we take to be truth. I have not recommended the abandonment of traditional science, but I do recommend that we equally credit the limitations of this method. By debunking the myths of scientific enterprise, we will find critical areas for new applications of that which is valuable in the scientific method and ways of integrating other patterns of knowing.

The fundamental question is not why we should question and challenge the myths of the scientific enterprise, but why not? Why not conceptualize the purposes and the goals of our research and theory in terms of the world that we want to create? Why not seriously value other ways of knowing? Why not value nursing and health? Why not identify actions, behaviors, and assumptions that we know to be consistent with health and behave as scientists in ways that are consistent with our vision? I believe that we are already beginning to do this; and if we choose to, we will increasingly focus our energies in this direction.

Acknowledgements

This article is adapted from a presentation given at the Research Day sponsored by Sigma Theta Tau Alpha Nu Chapter, Villanova University, Villanova, Pennsylvania, November 2, 1984. The author wishes to acknowledge the contributions of Charlene Eldridge Wheeler in conceptualizing the myths; of Barbara Carper in critiquing the methods for determining credibility of ethical, esthetic, and personal knowledge; and of the members of the Nursing Theory Think Tank for discussion that prompted the development of this article.

References

1. Carper B: Fundamental patterns of knowing in nursing. *Adv Nurs Sci* 1978;1:13-23.
2. Gorenberg B: The research tradition of nursing: An emerging issue. *Nurs Res* 1983;32:347-349.
3. Munhall PL: Nursing philosophy and nursing research: In apposition or opposition? *Nurs Res* 1982;31:176-177.
4. Newman M: *Theory Development in Nursing.* Philadelphia, FA Davis, 1979.
5. Smith MC: Research methodology: Epistemological considerations. *Image: The Journal of Nursing Scholarship* 1984;16:42-46.
6. Vredevoe DL: Curology: A basic science related to nursing. *Image: The Journal of Nursing Scholarship* 1984;16:89-92.
7. Webster G, Jacox A, Baldwin B: Nursing theory and the ghost of the receiving view, in Grace HK, McCloskey JC (eds): *Current Issues in Nursing.* Boston, Blackwell Scientific, 1981.
8. *Webster's New Collegiate Dictionary.* Springfield, Mass, GC Merriam, 1981.
9. Spender D: *Men's Studies Modified.* New York, Pergamon Press, 1981.
10. Spender D: *Man Made Language.* Boston, Routledge and Kegan Paul, 1980, pp 1-2.
11. Heide WS: *Feminism for the Health of it.* Ann Arbor, University Microfilms International, 1982.
12. Smith MJ: Transformation: A key to shaping nursing. *Image: The Journal of Nursing Scholarship* 1984;16:28-30.
13. Tinkle MB, Beaton JL: Towards a new view of science: Implications for nursing research. *Adv Nurs Sci* 1983;5:27-36.
14. Gilligan C: *In a Different Voice: Psychological Theory and Women's Development.* Cambridge, Harvard U Pr, 1982.
15. Munhall PL: Methodological fallacies: A critical self-appraisal. *Adv Nurs Sci* 1983;5:41-50.
16. Dock L: Foreign department. *Am J Nurs* 1915:15:666.

Baby Fae: The Unlearned Lesson

Kenneth P. Stoller, M.D.

On October 26, 1984, Dr. Leonard L. Bailey placed the heart of a baboon into the chest of Baby Fae, an infant born with a severe heart defect known as left hypoplastic heart. Baby Fae seemed to do well for a few days; then her body mounted a massive immunological attack on the foreign tissue and rejected the graft. Baby Fae's death came as no surprise to scientists and physicians familiar with the human immune system and with the scientific realities that preclude successful cross-species transplants.

Before the Baby Fae incident, Bailey, a surgeon at Loma Linda University Medical Center, spent almost a decade vainly pursuing research grants. His work in xenografts, largely unknown and unreviewed by other professionals, had not appeared in journals and was funded by Bailey himself and his colleagues.[1,2] During the seven years preceding the Baby Fae baboon transplant, he performed some 160 cross-species transplants, mostly on sheep and goats, none of whom survived more than 6 months. Although warned by a colleague at a medical conference that his research was too incomplete to risk using human subjects,[3] Bailey went ahead.

Baby Fae was not the first human to receive a primate xenograft. In a review of xenografts,[4] the Council of Scientific Affairs of the American Medical Association noted a rapid rejection of all baboon transplants to humans. Nevertheless, Bailey claimed that the problems of rejection could be overcome by the "immature" state of an infant's immune system. After the operation, immunologists from around the world pointed out that the part of the immune system that rejects unmatched transplants is fully mature at birth. Furthermore, there is no way to match baboon hearts to human recipients, because baboons have no antigens in common with human tissue.[5] Bailey has always maintained that Baby Fae's death was unrelated to the species of the organ "donor." An editorial in the *Journal of the American Medical Association* called Bailey's claim "wishful thinking."[5]

Bailey's use of baboons was somewhat surprising, given their relatively distant evolutionary relationship to humans compared to other primates. The reason came to light when the *Times* of London published an interview between Bailey and an Australian radio crew. The reporters had been forbidden to ask direct questions about the operation, so they queried Bailey on the issue of why he had chosen a baboon in view of the baboon's evolutionary distance from humans. Bailey replied, "Er, I find that difficult to answer. You see, I don't believe in evolution."[6] It is shocking that Bailey ignored basic biological concepts in formulating a life-threatening human experiment.

Often, ambitious surgeons wish to perform new, perhaps dangerous, experimental operations. In an effort to safeguard patients, institutional review boards must first give permission for any human experiment. In an unconscionable lapse of ethics, the review board of Loma Linda Medical Center failed to live up to its obligations -- they gave Bailey permission for five baboon-to-human transplant experiments, having no reports documenting that even heart allotransplantation in infancy is successful.[5] Furthermore, highly experimental procedures on children, such as a xenograft, require special permission from the Secretary of Health and Human Services.[7]

In addition to these institutional and federal safeguards that should have protected Baby Fae, California's Protection of Human Subjects in Medical Experimentation Act (PHSMEA) requires that if informed consent is given in behalf of another person, the experimental procedure must meet certain criteria. California's Health and Safety Code ~24175, subsection (e) states, "Informed consent given by a person other than the human subject shall only be for medical experiments related to maintaining or improving the health of the human subject or related to obtaining information about a pathological condition of the human subject."

Because Bailey did not look for a human heart donor and did not refer Baby Fae elsewhere for attempted surgical repair, the highly experimental transplant was both unethical and unlawful. Dr. William Norwood at the Children's Hospital in Boston has been repairing left hypoplastic hearts since 1979. The survival rate of the Norwood procedure is now as high as 75 percent. Nevertheless, Baby Fae's consent form read, "Temporizing operation to extend the lives of babies like yours by a few months have generally been unsuccessful. We believe heart transplantation may offer hope of life for your baby. Laboratory research at Loma Linda University over the past seven years, including over 150 heart transplants in newborn animals, suggest that long term survival with appropriate growth and development may be possible following heart transplantation during the first week of life."

Following considerable controversy over the Baby Fae transplant, the National Institutes of Health (NIH) appointed a special committee charged with reviewing the procedures used by the university to assure that Baby Fae's relatives gave proper informed consent. The committee did *not* deal with the scientific basis for transplanting a baboon heart into a human. The committee found several weaknesses in the consent procedure. Specifically, the committee concluded that possibility of "long term survival" had been overstated and the protocol did not include searching for or transplanting a human heart. The committee's report did not address why Loma Linda had not sought permission for this unprecedented experiment from the Secretary of Health and Human Services. Furthermore, it did not address the California law that should have prevented the experiment. (Perhaps the NIH committee was unaware of PHSMEA.)

Why hasn't Bailey been prosecuted? The San Bernandino District Attorney's office has officially stated that there are insufficient facts to support a felony prosecution. Unofficially, I was told that the highly technical nature of the case would likely overwhelm the court with conflicting medical opinions and therefore make a conviction unlikely. Furthermore, Bailey is considered a local hero. The office of the California State Attorney General, John K. Van de Kamp, has also maintained that insufficient facts are available to establish that a crime occurred.

The facts, however, suggest that Baby Fae was sacrificed to Leonard Bailey's career. Given the state of current medical knowledge, there was no doubt that Baby Fae would reject the baboon heart. Rules and laws designed to protect her were violated by those entrusted to uphold them. Professional ethics were considered to be of less importance than widespread publicity. The institutional review boards and law enforcement agencies responsible for protecting human subjects have virtually no accountability to the public, much less to the experimental subjects themselves.

References

1. Anon: Next please. *PCRM Update*, July-August, 1985.
2. Roe BB, Glaser RH: The lessons of the Baby Fae Case (letter). *The Wall Street Journal* Dec 24, 1984.
3. Mathews J: Colleague warned doctor before Baby Fae implant. *Washington Post*, 1984.
4. American Medical Association Council on Scientific Affairs: Xenografts: Review of the literature and current status. *JAMA* 1985;254:3353-3357.
5. Jonasson O, Hardy MA: The case of Baby Fae (letter). *JAMA* 1985;254:3358-3359.
6. Gould SJ: The heart of erminology: What has an abstruse debate over evolutionary logic got to do with Baby Fae? *Natural History* 1988;97:24.
7. Department of Health and Human Services: Final regulations amending basic HHS policy for the protection of human research subject. *Federal Register* 1981;465:8366-8392.

NIH Research Protocol for Silver Spring Monkeys: A Case of Scientific Misconduct

Neal D. Barnard, M.D., Roy Selby, M.D., Daniel N. Robinson, Ph.D., Gervasia M. Schreckenberg, Ph.D., Carol Van Petten, M.D.

Introduction

In 1981, police removed a group of monkeys, now known as the Silver Spring Monkeys, from the laboratory of psychologist Edward Taub, whose experiments were funded by the National Institutes of Health (NIH). Taub's research involved cutting the sensory nerves of monkeys' arms to see how well the monkeys could learn to use the numb limbs. Many of the animals mutilated their deadened limbs. The laboratory was grossly unsanitary, and there was a total absence of veterinary care. Taub was tried and convicted of animal cruelty, but his conviction was later overturned when an appellate court ruled that his federal funding exempted him from the provisions of Maryland's animal cruelty statute.

Thereafter, the monkeys were placed in the custody of the NIH and, later, the Delta Regional Primate Research Center. Many members of Congress have appealed to the NIH to transfer the animals to a primate sanctuary. The case has continued to be a source of conflict between the NIH on the one hand and animal protection groups and several Congressional offices on the other.

On or about July 1, 1988, a research protocol involving neurological experiments and euthanasia of the monkeys was sent to Congressmen Robert K. Dornan (R-CA) and Robert C. Smith (R-NH), and shortly thereafter to Congressman Charlie Rose (D-NC), all of whom have had a longstanding involvement with the case. The proposal was sent by William F. Raub, who was then NIH Deputy Director and is now Acting Director. Evidence strongly indicates that, in its content, its form, and the process by which it was proposed, the research protocol constitutes gross scientific misconduct and may have involved violations of regulations governing federally funded research. One of the proposal's aims was, apparently, to kill the animals who have been a source of poor public relations for the NIH.

This case is unique in several respects:

1. It appears that one motive behind the proposal was the intent to deceive one or more members of the U.S. Congress, particularly Robert

Dornan, Robert Smith, and Charlie Rose. Subsequently, attorneys for the NIH alluded to the proposed protocol in cases before the U.S. District Court for the Eastern District of Louisiana and the U.S. Court of Appeals for the Fifth Circuit, effectively using this proposal in such a manner that the courts would be deceived as to the scientific value of the animals in question.

2. The experiment has been conducted on only one monkey. Addressing this issue now would prevent the conduct of improper research of an invasive nature on the remaining animals.

3. Raub, who was then NIH Deputy Director and is currently Acting Director, has played a central role in this case. It is extraordinary that a high-ranking NIH official would offer such a research proposal, describe it as a "carefully" drawn experiment, and promote it in communications to Congressional offices. The circumstances surrounding the case suggest that, while Raub's advancement of the proposal to the Congressmen was rationalized by scientific arguments, its true aim had nothing to do with the specific area of scientific inquiry in question. This conclusion is supported both by the previous events in this case and the proposal's strikingly poor scientific quality and deficient form.

On October 2, 1985, Raub wrote a private letter to Joseph Vasapoli, Chief Executive Officer of the Institutes for Behavior Resources, owner of the monkeys. The letter, later obtained under the provisions of the Freedom of Information Act, stated that the NIH had no interest in using the animals for any research whatsoever and was anxious to be rid of them. Less than three years later, the research proposal was drafted and Raub sent it to Congressmen Dornan, Smith, and Rose. It states that the proposal would elicit "information that is potentially of great significance for alleviating suffering and advancing human health." The proposal was written, not by an extramural research institution, but by an anonymous author, and advanced to Congressional representatives by Raub. It is likely that former NIH Director James Wyngaarden had knowledge of the research proposal. It is, therefore, a case demanding an investigation of a scope beyond that required for cases of misconduct at extramural sites.

4. This case involves animals seized by police in Maryland in 1981. Their disposition has since been the subject of a prolonged series of lawsuits and Congressional actions, including requests signed by majorities of the U.S. Senate and House of Representatives that the animals be released from NIH custody.

5. Former NIH Director Wyngaarden has described the case of these animals as highly damaging to NIH's relationship with Congress. A resolu-

tion of the scientific fraud in this case is central to reestablishing a proper working relationship between Congress and those charged with the responsibility for carrying out federally funded research.

Circumstances Leading to Improper Proposal

The primates were seized by Montgomery County police from the Institute for Behavioral Research (IBR) in Silver Spring, Maryland in 1981. Thereafter, they were housed at an NIH facility in Poolesville, Maryland until 1986. On September 24, 1985, Joseph Vasapoli, Chief Executive Officer of IBR, which had been renamed the "Institutes for Behavior Resources," attempted to rid IBR of the animals. He wrote to Dr. Raub relinquishing ownership of the monkeys, because the original IBR investigator, Edward Taub, felt that the likelihood of his receiving funding to resume the research was "remote." On October 2, 1985, Dr. Raub responded:

> The NIH does not accept the proposal that we take ownership of them. We have no research protocols, either ongoing or planned, for which these animals are appropriate. As various NIH spokespersons have indicated from time to time, we wish to discontinue our temporary custody of the IBR monkeys as soon as possible.

The animals were transferred to Delta Primate Research Center in Covington, Louisiana in 1986. Five monkeys were later sent to the San Diego Zoo, and, although the remaining monkeys have been offered homes at two sanctuaries (Primarily Primates in Texas and Moorpark College in California), the NIH has refused to release them.

Related Experiments Advanced for Non-Scientific Aims

Although Raub's letter to Vasapoli clearly shows that the NIH had no interest in pursuing research with the monkeys, certain research proposals involving the animals were advanced by the NIH and scientific organizations soon thereafter, and were described as important experiments in briefings for Congressional officials. There is ample evidence that these proposals were not made to advance science, but to advance the NIH's interests in a lawsuit over custody of the monkeys and to prevail in related conflicts. Three research proposals, in fact, have been described to Congressional representatives in support of arguments for not relocating the monkeys. These three research proposals and the surrounding circumstances are briefly described below:

Proposal 1. Completion of Taub's original research. Taub lost his NIH grant following his arrest and the subsequent investigations, and IBR had many problems coming into compliance with applicable regulations. The NIH later approved an application from Dr. Taub to complete his research, but assigned it a low priority and did not fund it. NIH never sought any other investigator to complete the work. As noted above, Dr. Raub wrote to IBR in 1985 that the animals were not appropriate to any ongoing or planned NIH research. Raub specifically indicated to IBR that research on the animals was of no interest at NIH at that time, nor did he anticipate that that would change in the future.

In 1986, in response to a lawsuit brought by the International Primate Protection League and other animal protection groups to obtain custody of the monkeys so that they could be transferred to a primate sanctuary, several scientific organizations made a brief call for the completion of Taub's original research. The scientific organizations' principal concern was that if the court were to allow animal protection groups to bring suit over these animals, a precedent would be set recognizing that such groups have standing to sue over other animals involved in research.

Raub wrote to Congress on May 2, 1986, voicing this concern:

> The pending lawsuit has considerable national significance. If the courts rule that individuals or organizations that have no apparent rights of ownership with respect to particular laboratory animals have standing to bring litigation regarding their use or disposition, this could become a precedent for hundreds of such suits throughout the Nation. I am sure that you appreciate the adverse effect this could have on the progress of biomedical research.

Numerous scientific societies filed *amicus* briefs to influence the court to avoid establishing such a precedent. It is evident that representatives of several of these groups had been in direct or indirect contact with Raub, Wyngaarden, and others from the NIH, and that the animals' research value was advanced as a means to win the custody battle.

On April 30, 1986, less than seven months after Dr. Raub had stated that NIH had "no research protocols, either ongoing or planned, for which these animals are appropriate," a letter was sent to members of the U.S. Senate on the stationery of the Association of American Medical Colleges (AAMC) on behalf of 28 other organizations "whose members are heavily engaged in biomedical and behavioral research and health care." The letter was sent in anticipation of oral arguments before the U.S. Court of Appeals for the

Fourth Circuit, which were scheduled for May 8. Although the letter contains non-specific praise for the idea of completing Taub's original research protocol, its motivation was clearly to prevent the plaintiffs from achieving any precedent-setting decision. First, representatives of the signatory organizations verbally stated that this was their motivation, as is detailed below. Second, these groups stopped promoting the research as soon as the court case ended. Third, the letter's text is explicit in this regard:

> The precedent that would be established by acceding to their demands would have a disruptive effect on both the research and academic communities and would severely damage the longstanding, interdependent relationship between the federal government and those communities.

At that time, one author of the present critique (Dr. Barnard) called representatives of a number of the groups listed as signatories to that letter. Their statements clearly indicate that their involvement in the court proceedings stemmed from a desire to cooperate with other scientific organizations in an attempt to fight the establishment of a legal precedent, rather than from an interest in specific research involving these animals. Several of these representatives stated that they had been told that Taub's original research had merit and should be completed, but none had detailed knowledge of the research. Several had been told by Raub or Wyngaarden that the animals could not be adequately cared for at a sanctuary. Quotations from a number of these representatives follow. They demonstrate that expressed interest in the research in question was not genuine, but was aimed at the issue of legal standing which might, if recognized by the courts, later impact on their own interests. In addition, they show the degree of pressure felt by the NIH and the scientific organizations involved in the case. This pressure appears to have ultimately led to improper research proposals. Here, listed by organization, are some statements made by individual representatives:

The Shock Society: "[We] just wanted to support the principle to show solidarity with our colleagues. I haven't looked over the protocols. The principle is not giving in to terrorist groups or groups that are not accredited."

The American Psychiatric Association: "The issue has to do with protecting NIH from getting involved with this stuff. NIH wound up with these monkeys. They're an incidental kind of thing. It's really an issue of -- we strongly support research. . . . We have usually stood with other research organizations. . . . I'm not an expert on this. . . . I respect Bill Raub. NIH must have a plan for using them."

The American Diabetes Association: "The Foundation for Biomedical Research and AAMC drafted the letter. It was our judgment that it was important enough to sign on to . . . . The overriding issue is that animal rights groups should not be granted standing. Animal rights groups could impede or halt research."

The Association of American Medical Colleges: "There is a principle at stake. If PETA (People for the Ethical Treatment of Animals) is able through the political process to establish the ability to influence the outcome of something of this nature, we're in for some real trouble."

The Massachusetts General Hospital: "We signed on because we are concerned about the general protection of the use of animals in research. I was not familiar with this research before this issue came up."

The Pharmaceutical Manufacturers Association: "The major reason [we signed on to the AAMC letter] was the problem of standing that these groups might obtain if they win the court case on these animals. That's our primary concern."

The American College of Surgeons: "We have to go along with what we're advised to do. We only know what we're told."

The Association of Academic Health Centers: "[We are] in support of thc general issue and the need for animals in research. We have no specific interest in the animals."

The Association of American Universities: "We're concerned about the impact on research. . . . We heard that some of the animals could not be properly cared for at Primarily Primates. . . . Bill Raub told me that last Friday."

The National Association of State Universities and Land-Grant Colleges: "We have people committed to the notion that, for a great deal of research, animals are necessary. . . . Eight of those monkeys can't be moved. They received very radical surgery. They're very fragile. I'm not saying the controls couldn't be moved. I stood with Wyngaarden in a corner at a party last week on the Hill. I asked him, because I'd heard from two other sources at NIH that they couldn't be moved. He says they need daily veterinary care. He told me the first time in a corner, and the second time at a meeting. The second time, I asked him at a meeting -- an impromptu thing. We have an ad hoc group on biomedical research to get money for ADAMHA. He gave us a briefing at the Hill. They did not have, to his understanding, the good solid veterinary care that those animals would need on a daily basis. . . . I've heard Bill Raub and others at NIH say they have all the paper work done by Taub and that follow-up work is entirely possible.

We don't have any thought whatsoever on that."

The National Foundation for Infectious Diseases: "[We are interested] strictly in the generic issue, that's all."

The American Council on Education: "We're really concerned with the litigation more than anything else."

The American Federation for Clinical Research: "We're all concerned about the precedent that this would set. We're not concerned about the 15, but animals in general. . . . The information (gained by completing Taub's original research protocol) could be quite valuable." When asked how, the representative quoted a brief from the National Association for Biomedical Research, and indicated that she had no specific or independent knowledge of the research.

The American Society for Microbiology: "The concern is for the precedent. This could set a precedent for animal activists to make demands."

It is impossible to avoid the conclusion that the idea of completing Taub's original research was advanced, not for scientific aims, but to assist NIH's effort in the lawsuit and the continuing public relations battle. Moreover, there is an apparent acceptance of the practice of proposing and advocating experiments in order to affect a court decision and to create an impression in federal legislators.

The interest in Taub's original research waned almost immediately. On June 13, 1986, in a briefing to Congress, Dr. Wyngaarden stated that NIH had again abandoned interest in the original research except for necropsies of the animals after their natural deaths. The medical organizations which were politically active in the issue stopped promoting Taub's original research as soon as the court decided that the animal protection groups did not have standing to sue.

Proposal 2: Resocialization research. The second research area, proposed by Dr. Wyngaarden in his June 13, 1986 Congressional briefing, was primate resocialization. Since the monkeys had been in prolonged isolation and could perhaps be put into groups, Wyngaarden described resocialization process as a potentially valuable field of study. In a letter to Congressman Smith four days earlier, Wyngaarden has written of this line of research with particular emphasis on a monkey with bilaterally deafferented limbs:

> The knowledge gained from this process could have the benefits of contributing to better understanding of primate behavior in group situations and thereby advance both animal care and conservation efforts.. . . The remaining primate, an animal with both forelimbs disabled, will be cared for individually. The nature and extent of its use of disabled limbs will be

> studied through systematic observations. The knowledge gained could contribute to better understanding of the possibility for recovery from this type of disability.

This small group of animals could certainly not overshadow the social processes of the other 3,000 primates at Delta and numerous investigators' years of research on primate social processes. The suggestion of "resocialization research" made by the head of the NIH had no obvious connection to genuine significant research interests and appears to have been advanced for public relations purposes, aimed at Congressional offices.

No detailed proposals were ever offered for this research. The control monkeys were later put into groups at the San Diego Zoo, and the idea of research on resocialization of the deafferented monkeys appears to have been abandoned. In part, this may be because the NIH's assessments of the monkeys' health have changed over time, as is discussed below. Wyngaarden's credibility on this issue came even more into question at that time, because of other promises he made: He stated that the monkeys would not be moved without notification of the parties involved in the litigation and that they would not be relocated without being surgically prepared, i.e., having their deafferented arms amputated. But only ten days after the Congressional briefing, on June 23, 1986, the animals were secretly loaded into trucks and transferred to Delta without prior notification and without any surgical preparation.

Proposal 3: Neurological experiments and euthanasia. The NIH protocol sent to Congressmen Dornan and Smith on July 1, 1988 was the third research proposal involving the animals since Taub's trial.

The NIH appears to have felt continuing pressure to make a case for the monkeys' research value. In April and May of 1986, a majority of the U.S. Senate signed a letter to Dr. Wyngaarden asking that the monkeys be transferred to a sanctuary. A majority of the House of Representatives signed a similar letter. Editorials calling for the monkeys' release appeared in many newspapers. Although the standing issue is over, the NIH has remained at odds with animal protection groups and several Congressional offices regarding the case. Wyngaarden has described the case of these animals as highly damaging to the NIH and its relationship with Congress, and a threat to its financial support. In Science and Government Report, May 15, 1989, Wyngaarden stated:

> We have had probably no single more enervating case than the Silver Spring monkey case. It was here when I arrived and it will be here when I leave.

> . . . [Because of this and other controversies] some of our strong backers on the House Appropriations Committee say it's a little harder each year to get this sort of kneejerk response supporting the NIH budget from the rest of the Congress. They have to work harder at selling their colleagues, not within the Subcommittee, but sometimes within the full Committee, and certainly within the Congress as a whole. All of these issues have made it a little more difficult to get the kind of broad, unquestioned backing for the NIH that it once had.

Delta's director, Peter Gerone, called for "scientists to unite and become proactive on animal issues in order to resist the mounting pressure exerted by animal rights activists," whom Gerone described as "fanatics" and "misanthropes."[1] The American Medical Association, the Massachusetts Society for Medical Research, and some government officials have developed detailed proposals for battling animal protection groups that have called for an uncompromising stand. It appears that Gerone and NIH officials have viewed releasing the animals as tantamount to surrender to animal protection groups. Given the atmosphere in the scientific community, NIH officials appear to have attempted to make a case for killing the animals and/or using them in research, rather than yield to pressure to release them.

Violation of Assurances to Congress

Invasive experiments on these animals violate a clear agreement between the NIH and Congress. In a June 9, 1986 letter to Congressman Robert C. Smith, NIH Director James Wyngaarden wrote, "These animals will not undergo invasive procedures for research purposes." The definition of "invasive" in *Dorland's Medical Dictionary*, 26th Edition, is as follows: "Involving puncture or incision of the skin or insertion of an instrument or foreign material into the body." In hearings before a subcommittee of the House Appropriations Committee, Wyngaarden repeated, "No invasive procedures will be performed on the animals."

On July 10, 1986, Assistant Secretary for Health Robert E. Windom wrote, "The Delta Center has agreed to house the animals, under very strict conditions, including that they will not be used for any further invasive research."

In a January 6, 1987 letter, Tulane President Eamon M. Kelly wrote, "We have publicly stated that the Center will not do any invasive research on the animals, and we intend to abide by that statement."

A January 8, 1987 Fact Sheet from NIH stated, "No further invasive research will be done on the animals."

In an August 15, 1986 letter to a concerned citizen, Gerone wrote:

> Non-invasive research would be research that does not require infecting, cutting, inoculating or otherwise invading the animal's body. This should not be construed to mean, however, that we would not invade the animal's body for medical purposes. We intend to take whatever means are indicated to protect the health of the animals. Your questions imply that. . . . we can't be trusted to do what we say we're going to do. I resent that. I would not make public statements that our only concern is for the welfare of the animals and then turn around and use them experimentally.

In a November 20, 1986 letter to Congresswoman Boggs, Gerone wrote, "Please assure your constituents that we do not intend to do any research on these animals." Boggs then used this assurance as the basis for responding to concerned constituents.

Yet the experiment, carried out January 14, 1990, was clearly invasive. Its protocol -- the third proposed by the NIH -- involved cutting the scalp, skull, and meninges and passing electrodes into the brain. Despite its public assurances that the monkeys would not be subjected to further invasive research, Gerone was intermittently present as the experiment was performed. He had, in fact, listed himself as the experiment's principal investigator when Delta's animal care committee considered and approved the experiment.

Invasiveness is an important issue for two reasons:

(1) Manipulating the time frame of "humane" euthanasia. The decision to euthanize is to be based on humane considerations, not the desire to facilitate an experiment. Clearly, however, the experiment affected the decision to euthanize. In late December, Delta officials planned to begin the experiment on one monkey (Billy) on the assumption that they could obtain permission from the other parties in the pending lawsuit. They stated that although they believed euthanasia was necessary, they wished to delay it several days in order to bring in investigators from Nashville. This arrangement fell apart when plaintiffs refused to agree. On January 14, 1990, Gerone stated that euthanasia should occur that day, because if Billy were to die at night, the experimental results would be lost.

It should be noted that the procedure is to be done only when an individual animal requires euthanasia for humane reasons, e.g., severe, intractable pain. In such a case, delaying euthanasia in order to assemble a group of investigators and bring them to the site where the procedures are to take place violates NIH assurances concerning these monkeys. Delays in scheduling and transportation would be expected, given the number of investigators involved and the distance they presumably travel. The protocol also overlooks the fact that some of the animals may not require euthanasia. There is no provision for the animals to be allowed to die naturally.

(2) Pain. The protocol is intended to be implemented when each animal is so debilitated that euthanasia is required. At that point, anesthesia is risky for the animal. Those administering anesthesia might keep it too light, since maintaining deep anesthesia could inadvertently kill the subject and defeat the four-hour experiment. Gerone and Dr. Ratterree, a Delta veterinarian, stated in a phone conversation during the hearing before Judge Sporkin on January 14, 1990 that Billy would not be able to tolerate one hour of anesthesia for the placement of a feeding tube, yet it was necessary that he withstand four hours of anesthesia for the experiment.

The Euthanasia Question

The NIH protocol included both euthanasia of the monkeys and various neurological measurements. According to Raub, the protocol was to be used when euthanasia was required for humane reasons. A review of the various examinations of the animals reveals that Raub and Delta officials have attempted to make a case for euthanasia on tenuous grounds.

On October 1, 1986, two physicians, Douglas M. Koltun and Joseph J. Biundo, examined the monkeys and reported their findings. They noted abnormalities in the physical examinations and X-rays, most of which related to the condition of the deafferented limbs. They were impressed that one monkey, Nero, had undergone an amputation of his deafferented limb and was doing quite well:

> This animal appeared to reach for food aggressively with his right hand and had no trouble in attempts to manipulate the food. Evaluation when under anesthesia showed that the skin of the left upper extremity/shoulder region was well healed and the patient appeared to have had the amputation just distal to the humeral head.

They recommended that amputation of the deafferented limbs be considered for all the monkeys except Billy, who was bilaterally deafferented, and was killed in the course of the experiment on January 14, 1990. They did not recommend euthanasia for any of the monkeys. In a telephone conversation with Dr. Barnard on February 16, 1987, Dr. Koltun confirmed that no animal appeared to be in any pain, and that amputation of the deafferented limbs would probably allow them to be safely resocialized. He again confirmed that euthanasia was not indicated. Dr. Koltun stated, "Judging from my impression of Nero, I thought it likely that they'd be able to do well with an amputated arm."

On December 3, 1986, Gerone convened a four-member "Ad Hoc Committee for the Resocialization Plan of the Silver Spring Monkeys" to make recommendations regarding the animals. The committee was given the report of Drs. Koltun and Biundo, and descriptions of the animals' physical status by Delta veterinarians Robert Wolf and Edwin Watson. Committee members did not conduct physical examinations on the animals. A letter from Raub to People for the Ethical Treatment of Animals, dated April 20, 1987, indicates that he had been in close touch with the committee throughout the period in which the report was generated.

In marked contrast to the medical findings of Drs. Koltun and Biundo, the Committee recommended euthanasia for all the deafferented animals as the preferred course of action. Although the physicians' examination did not note evidence of pain and Dr. Koltun specifically reported that none of the animals seemed to be in any pain, and despite the positive results from Nero's amputation, the Ad Hoc Committee reported that the animals were probably in pain which could not be relieved by amputation. No rationale was given for this judgment. In fact, the committee report noted that "Visual inspection of the animals revealed no obvious behavioral pathologies" that might indicate pain. In studies of groups of humans who have suffered deafferentation, pain is the exception, rather than the rule.[2] Moreover, nowhere in the Ad Hoc Committee report or any other report generated in any aspect of this case is there any mention of any effort to alleviate pain. There is no mention that pain medications have been used, or even considered. This raises questions as to whether the "pain" mentioned by Wolf, Watson, and others was, in fact, present and whether the goal of those recommending euthanasia was truly pain relief.

In the event that euthanasia was rejected, the Ad Hoc Committee recommended amputation of affected limbs and resocialization. Other options were also suggested.

Three months later, a memorandum written at the American Physiological Society (APS) revealed what appears to be the context in which the euthanasia decision was made. The memo, dated March 17, 1987, indicates that extensive discussions occurred between APS, Tulane University (of which Delta is a part), the Institutes for Behavior Resources, the Society for Neuroscience, and the American Psychological Association, and that these groups had developed a plan to deal with the case. The plan included private payments to Tulane, which could be reduced and more easily arranged if the deafferented monkeys were killed. The memo stated:

> The scientific community has negotiated with IBR and governmental agencies a possible resolution to which everyone (except the animal rights advocates who want the monkeys given to them) has given an agreement to the general details. PROPOSED AGREEMENT -- IBR gives title to the monkeys to Tulane University, thus freeing NIH from any responsibility as to the future of these animals. IBR pays NIH $16,000 owed for the monkeys' feed bill. (This is a possible snag as IBR in the past has refused to pay the bill. However, we have been told that there is a change of heart within IBR on this issue). . . . Tulane wants an endowment so neither state nor federal funds are involved.
>
> If all 14 monkeys were to be maintained for the normal life expectancies, it has been calculated that $95,000 would have to be raised. With the treated animals to be euthanized it has been estimated that $35,000 to $50,000 needs to be raised.
>
> Proposal to APS [American Physiological Society] -- Fred King, director of the Yerkes Regional Primate Center in Atlanta, has been discussing with the Society for Neurosciences and the American Psychological Association the need to raise the funds to endow the lifetime care for the monkeys. Both organizations have agreed to do it if APS would be the third member.
>
> Neurosciences, APA, and APS are the three organizations that have been involved directly in this seemingly never-ending episode, largely because Dr. Ed Taub, who was doing the research on the monkeys, is a member of all three organizations.

Tulane, then, would relieve the NIH of its longstanding public relations problem in exchange for payments from private sources. If the deafferented animals were killed, the payments could be reduced by $45,000-60,000. The required sum would then be considerably easier to raise. Also, the living symbols of federally funded cruelty would no longer exist.

On June 26, 1987, Janis Ott Joslin, a veterinarian, examined the monkeys at the request of the Louisiana Society for the Prevention of Cruelty to Animals (LSPCA). How this group made a liaison with Delta is unclear. Dr. Joslin reported that the monkeys were active, alert, and in generally good health. She reported that she had been cautioned by Delta's Wolf and Watson that the animals may be experiencing "phantom pain" in their deafferented limbs that amputations would not alleviate, that the amputation sites might not heal, and that putting the animals into larger enclosures might lead to falls and trauma. Joslin's report provided no basis for Wolf's and Watson's opinions.

Dr. Joslin recommended that limb amputation and resocialization be considered on an individual basis. She did not report evidence of pain except for raising the possibility of pain for Billy, the double-deafferented monkey, and did not call for euthanasia of any of the animals, except for asking that it be considered for Billy.

Three days later, on June 29, 1987, Gary L. Frazell of the Louisiana SPCA issued a report on his Delta visit, which consisted of viewing the animals and being told by Wolf and Watson of their condition. Frazell, who is not a physician, veterinarian, or scientist, lacked the expertise to evaluate the animals independently and was not given the chance to do so. His conclusions were explicitly based on what those conducting his visit had told him. Wolf and Watson evidently used their speculations regarding "phantom pain" to encourage Frazell to recommend euthanasia for all the animals. He wrote:

> Both Dr. Wolf and Dr. Watson . . . demonstrated through the use of x-rays that the spinal columns of these monkeys had, in varying degrees, deteriorated markedly. They expressed their belief that because of spinal deterioration several or possibly all of the eight monkeys are experiencing continual pain. On the assumption that this information is well founded I recommend that the eight monkeys be euthanized without further delay.

A seven-member panel wrote an Assessment of and Recommendations for "the Silver Spring Monkeys" on March 16-18, 1988. The panel recommended that two animals be killed and that three possibly be resocialized. The panel also concluded that four of the monkeys did not require euthanasia but were poor candidates for resocialization. The report praised Delta's staff and, curiously, contained unattributed language that was nearly identical to that contained in the anonymous NIH research protocol. For example, the first paragraph on page six of the panel report is nearly identical to the first paragraph of the protocol section "Background of the Scientific Problem." The second paragraph of the panel report and the protocol are also strikingly similar, strongly suggesting that the two were not drafted independently. The panel report also made an impassioned plea for neurological research on the animals.

Although euthanasia was recommended for two of the monkeys, there are no clinical findings that provide a rationale for this. A variety of skeletal abnormalities are present in these monkeys (joint luxation, scoliosis, lordosis, hypertrophic spondylitis, and joint fusion). The panel, however, did not conclude that these abnormalities caused the animals pain or discomfort, and there is no mention of "phantom limb pain." These same abnormalities are common in humans and do not, in and of themselves, indicate an unacceptable degree of pain.

A page of hand-written notes from the office of Adrian Morrison, a University of Pennsylvania veterinarian who has long been involved in the Silver Spring Monkeys case, indicates that the decision to kill all the animals at once was modified in order to avoid attracting protests from animal rights groups. These notes state, "Euthanize them . . . then decided to euth 2 right away and delay others . . . so PETA wouldn't descend."

An additional concern affecting the decision to kill rather than release the animals was revealed in a November 14, 1988 letter to Raub from panel member Douglas Bowden, Director of the Regional Primate Research Center at the University of Washington. In his letter to Raub, Bowden advised against relocating the monkeys to a private facility. In spite of the public relations cost of killing a "surplus animal," Bowden wrote:

> (It) would be incalculably higher, however, were NIH to set a precedent whereby any lesioned animal from a nonterminal research project becomes an automatic candidate for transfer to a PETA surrogate for nonresearch purposes.
>
> Our experience illustrates the kind of harassment and media event that is likely to occur repeatedly throughout the country if NIH establishes a precedent that lesioned research animals be sold or donated for nonscientific purposes. Every surplus lesioned animal in which PETA or any other anti-research organization registers an interest would become the potential subject of a bitter and protracted public debate. . . . I do not know the risk-benefit analysis of the consequences of a policy reversal for NIH per se. But for the US biomedical research community as a whole, it would be disastrous.

It is uncertain to what extent Bowden's opinions regarding the "disastrous" consequences of releasing the monkeys affected his behavior on the panel, but it is clearly inappropriate to consider the panel independent or objective.

An additional problem with the panel report is its inexplicable neglect of the possibility of amputation of the damaged limbs, which would allow the animals to be resocialized. In the panel report, potential damage to the deafferented limb appears to be the major reason for euthanasia and for avoiding resocialization efforts. Given that the report by Drs. Koltun and Biundo recommending amputation was made available to the panel, why wasn't amputation discussed? Also, the report indicates that individual housing was required because monkeys grouped together might fight; however, the control monkeys, also males, are group-housed at the San Diego

Zoo and have done well in that arrangement. In summary, it appears that the panel was far from objective on the most pressing questions regarding the animals' fate.

On September 26, 1988, James Peddie, D.V.M. and Gary L. Wilson, Director of the Exotic Animal Training and Management Program of Moorpark College, evaluated the monkeys and combined their findings with those of Donald Lindburg, Ph.D. of the San Diego Zoo, who had served on the panel of March 16-18, 1988. It was concluded that the monkeys could be safely transported to Moorpark and cared for there, with the exception of Paul, who was infected with the Herpes B virus and who has since died.

In response to these recommendations, Raub wrote a letter to Wilson at Moorpark, expressing grave disappointment:

> I am dismayed at your conclusion that Moorpark College could safely move and provide adequate care for seven of the eight experimentally disabled Silver Spring monkeys. The report is inaccurate, incomplete, and otherwise seriously misleading for the uninitiated reader. The egregious misrepresentation of Dr. Donald Lindburg's role and views is particularly distressing and will leave you no credibility. . . . I need a . . . commitment from you . . . to make decisions strictly on the basis of the pertinent facts and informed opinion. For you and I to do otherwise is to become pawns for those who desperately seek to devalue the opinions and impugn the integrity of the several experts whose wise counsel has guided the NIH, the Delta Center, and the San Diego Zoo to date in caring for the monkeys.

Raub then wrote to Congressman Smith of his dismay over Wilson's report and stated:

> With respect to the most seriously disabled monkeys, we have deferred the euthanasia decision since July at your and Mr. Dornan's request. However, further delay no longer is tenable. Consultants with superb credentials and experience, who have studied these monkeys' conditions thoroughly, have given us clear-cut guidance on this matter. To keep the three most disabled monkeys alive for any significant additional time would constitute animal cruelty in our judgment.

Raub's letter is striking both in its description of the previous poorly supported euthanasia recommendations as "clear-cut guidance," and in Raub's statement against what he called "animal cruelty." Raub has not championed the humane treatment of animals in the past. Regarding Raub's letter, Wilson responded to Congressman Smith:

> I was surprised by Dr. Raub's reaction to our evaluation of the Silver Spring monkeys. It seems he is quite unaware of Dr. Lindburg's position regarding these animals. Dr. Lindburg, Dr. Peddie, and myself all have come to the same conclusion, i.e., these animals are not in as poor condition as previous evaluations have indicated. . . . Dr. Peddie, in the course of treating traumatized animals, encounters quite similar problems routinely in his clinical practice and does not think of these problems as being that severe and unmanageable. . . . I was looking for signs the animals were suffering from either the deafferentation procedure or their long period of confinement. I was surprised at how well they appear to be doing. . . . I would only consider the Silver Spring monkeys candidates for euthanasia if there is no possibility for improving the quality of their life.

It is evident that Raub and Delta officials have called for euthanasia in the absence of a clear rationale. Their recommendation has been disputed by other experts who have examined the monkeys both before and after the committee reports Raub has cited.

Raub has been joined in this call for euthanasia by some of the same organizations which, in 1986, briefly called for the completion of Taub's original research as a means of preventing animal groups from gaining standing in court. The National Association for Biomedical Research, the Federation of American Societies for Experimental Biology, and other organizations have made uncharacteristic pleas for euthanasia as the "humane" course for the animals. None of these groups has a history of advocacy for the humane treatment of animals. Indeed, they have frequently been on record opposing animal protection legislation. It is difficult to avoid the conclusion that the call for euthanasia is intended to serve self-interest. As part of the euthanasia plan, Raub advanced the third experimental protocol.

Delta's Role

As indicated above, Tulane University, which is the university affiliate of Delta, was actively involved in formulating a plan to relieve the NIH of the monkeys and the associated public relations problems in exchange for payments to be arranged by scientific organizations, particularly those to which Edward Taub, the original experimenter, belonged.

An additional part of the controversy concerns the care offered at Delta. The panel convened at Delta on March 16-18, 1988 had great praise for the care the animals have received at Delta. Animal protection groups, however, have been concerned about Delta's high rate of accidental deaths prior to the monkeys' arrival and the deaths of two of the deafferented monkeys since arriving at Delta. One presumably died of a pulmonary infection resulting from aspiration during feeding. The other died after a long illness for which the Delta veterinarians were never able to arrive at a diagnosis. It has been reported that no veterinarian was in attendance at the time that this monkey died and that, although tissue samples were taken, the body was incinerated without an examination by independent veterinarians. The NIH protocol was not used at that time.

A November, 1989 report on the monkeys' condition released by the NIH revealed that several were self-mutilating, presumably due to stress and to the NIH's failure to remove their flail arms. Several had dermatologic conditions and intestinal infections due to living in cramped individual cages in which they were continually exposed to their own wastes. All of these conditions would be responsive to proper care.

Peter Gerone, Delta's director, has been consistently active regarding the case's public relations aspects. On April 21, 1989, Gerone complained to James W. Glosser, Administrator of the Animal and Plant Health Inspection Service (APHIS) of the U.S. Department of Agriculture (USDA), that a federal inspection report had noted deficiencies in conditions at Delta. While Gerone admitted that the violations were accurately noted, he went so far as to suggest that the inspectors should have violated federal law by omitting these failures from their written report in order to avoid damaging Delta's reputation. Gerone wrote:

> If I may make a point, let's assume that I am an antivivisectionist and I request this report through the Freedom of Information Act. I could write the following headline:
> "The Delta Regional Primate Research Center of Tulane University, home of the Silver Spring monkeys, was recently cited for 5 deficiencies in an unscheduled visit by a USDA veterinarian. They were given 30 days in which to correct these deficiencies."
> That would be a perfectly true statement and would have a very damaging effect on what is an excellent, world-class primate research facility. The point I am making is that USDA, without intending to do so, is playing into the hands of the animal rights/antivivisectionists. . . . Someone else mentioned that the USDA and APHIS are our "friends" in this fight over the use of animals in research. . . . [I]f these are our friends, we don't need any enemies! . . . We would not quarrel with any of the points that were made by the inspector. He could have told us about them and we would have corrected them immediately. What I do quarrel with is having these stated in writing and giving us a written ultimatum to correct them in 30 days. . . . I am convinced that, if you are trying to placate the animal rights

> activists by nit-picking inspections, you are engaged in an exercise in futility, and you will only serve to do us irreparable harm.

Gerone then offered to buy Glosser a ticket to New Orleans to speak about the issue further. Gerone seems to have forgotten that federal law mandates written reports of inspections. On August 7, 1989, Gerone played a principal role (chair of fund-raising and membership) in an organizational meeting of the Foundation for Animal Use in Society, with the explicit intention of soliciting the involvement of the fur industry, rodeos, hunting and trapping groups, livestock producers, meat processors, auction barns, and animal research groups in a "proactive" effort to protect their interests. Notes from the meeting show that the Society was to be described to the public as "an animal welfare organization."

Gerone has played an active role in the Silver Spring Monkey case since the monkeys were moved to his facility. In an application to Delta's Institutional Animal Care and Use Committee asking approval of the new NIH experiment, Gerone listed himself as Principal Investigator, although he has no relevant experience and played no evident role in drafting the experiment.

Litigation in the case continues. When the NIH announced its intention to kill three of the animals and carry out the euthanasia/research protocol, the International Primate Protection League and other groups filed suit in Louisiana State Court to prevent the NIH from doing so. The court issued a temporary restraining order blocking the NIH from harming or killing the animals. The NIH successfully sought to have the case moved to Federal District Court, which upheld the restraining order. Currently, the NIH is appealing to the U.S. Court of Appeals for the 5th Circuit. The temporary restraining order was voided on January 11, 1990, so that Billy could be experimented on, then euthanized. On January 12, a new restraining order was issued in response to a lawsuit filed by Physicians Committee for Responsible Medicine. On January 14, NIH attorneys submitted a declaration from Peter Gerone to the Court to the effect that Billy was about to die, and that the experiment should be conducted at once in order to avoid losing valuable data. The order was again voided; that evening, Billy was experimented on and killed.

Scientific Misconduct in NIH Protocol

The following sections review evidence of misconduct in the NIH protocol.

Definition of Scientific Misconduct

Scientific misconduct is investigated by the NIH's Office of Scientific Integrity (OSI) as well as the Office of Scientific Integrity Review (OSIR) in the Office of the Assistant Secretary of Health, Department of Health and Human Services. According to OSIR Director Lyle W. Bivens, "misconduct in science" is defined in Title 42, part 50 of the Code of Federal Regulations as "fabrication, falsification, plagiarism, or other practices that seriously deviate from those that are commonly accepted within the scientific community for proposing, conducting or reporting research."

Evidence suggests that serious and willful misconduct was involved in the writing and advancement of the NIH protocol. It appears that among the motives behind this fraudulent proposal was the intent to deceive members of Congress; the proposal also had the effect of deceiving judges in federal court.

Representation of the NIH Protocol as Duly Authorized Research

In his July 1, 1988 letter, Raub represented the NIH protocol to Congressman Dornan as a "carefully" drawn plan that would be carried out in conjunction with euthanasia. Raub's letter stated:

> Staff of the Department of Health and Human Services (HHS) and collaborators therefore have prepared a plan for the euthanasia (Enclosure B). This plan is drawn carefully to ensure due recognition of both the special protected status of the animals and the unique neurological information they can provide with respect to improved treatment for human victims of stroke or spinal cord injury.

Documents submitted to the U.S. Court of Appeals for the Fifth Circuit by attorneys for the NIH show that the NIH encouraged the court to believe that a properly designed and approved research protocol existed. The apparent motivation was a desire to prevail in a legal proceeding over the fate of the monkeys in question. The NIH had previously indicated its plan to kill three of the animals, but the plan was blocked by a temporary restraining order. When the NIH's appeal to the U.S. District Court for the Eastern District of Louisiana was heard, Thomas Watson, representing NIH, stated:

> First of all, the NIH does have an interest in this case, obviously, Your

> Honor, and that's to fulfill its mission which is to conduct research on these monkeys. In that proceeding, it was clear that the judge had been made to believe that experiments were to be conducted on the animals, as indicated by the statement of the Court: From what I understand, they will be put to death or experiments will be continued on them at the time they are being put to death.

In documents submitted to the U.S. Court of Appeals for the Fifth Circuit in July, 1989, the Brief for the Appellant (NIH) calls the protocol "important research procedures" in its Request for Oral Argument:

> The District Court issued a preliminary injunction that bars NIH from euthanizing three research monkeys and from carrying out certain important research procedures on the monkeys in a nonpainful manner during the euthanasia process.

On page 13 of the Brief, NIH attorneys stated:

> Through humane, nonpainful procedures that would be conducted as part of and following the euthanasia procedure involving deep surgical anaesthesia, NIH hopes to gain important knowledge that may lead to substantial improvements in rehabilitation therapy for individuals who have suffered brain or spinal cord damage.

On page 15 and again on page 37, the protocol is represented to the Court as "important research."

On September 29, 1989, NIH attorneys requested expedited oral argument in the court case, stating, "NIH has been prevented from carrying out its plans to conduct important medical research on certain experimental monkeys because of a temporary restraining order issued on January 5, 1989."

In arguments in federal court on January 10, NIH attorneys used arguments of the experiment's scientific value in order to have the temporary restraining order voided for one monkey, Billy. They stated that the experiment related to rehabilitation and pharmaceutical treatments, when in fact it does not:

> The medical information NIH will obtain from those procedures is of the utmost significance, relating as it does to the rehabilitation therapy and pharmaceutical treatment of humans who have sustained brain or spinal cord damage. . . . If the preliminary injunction is not lifted in time for NIH and Tulane to conduct the painless research described in the attached declarations, the answers to the human tragedy of quadriplegia and paraplegia,

among other such conditions, may remain locked in Billy's brain forever.

Evidently, no other, more detailed protocol for the experiment was submitted for approval. On October 19, 1989, Congressman Smith wrote to Raub asking "(1) whether NIH plans to adhere to the [July 1988] provisions planned for these animals; and (2) do any other documents exist regarding the future use of these animals?" Raub responded on November 17: "the July 1988 protocol remains our intent. Absent judicial constraints, we would effect that procedure immediately for at least three of the monkeys." On January 10, 1990, NIH attorneys submitted the protocol to the U.S. District Court for the Eastern District of Louisiana, indicating their wish to carry out its provisions. NIH attorneys reportedly stated in federal court in Louisiana that no other protocol exists. In U.S. District Court for the District of Columbia on January 12, 1990, NIH attorneys stated that no more finished document had ever been written.

NIH Representatives clearly wished federal officials to believe that the July 1988 document represented properly designed research that should be carried out without further amendments or approvals.

Critique of Protocol

The protocol's content is grossly deviant from accepted scientific norms in several respects. The report consists of five main sections: "Introduction," "Background of the Scientific Problem," "Goals," "Protocol for Euthanasia and Post-Mortem Analysis of Tissues," and "Summary."

Improprieties are noted below in two categories: content and administrative procedures. This separation is somewhat artificial. For example, the absence of an identified principal investigator on the original protocol is a deficiency of both content and procedure. To avoid redundancy, however, each deficiency was assigned to only one category.

Critique of Protocol: Content

The four-and-one-half-page document is markedly shorter than that of typical research protocols, which are comprehensive documents that may reach hundreds of pages in length. There are glaring omissions:

1. No principal investigator is listed. Research proposals are normally submitted by a principal investigator and one or more co-investigators whose qualifications are subjected to scrutiny by the inclusion of their curricula vitae. The NIH protocol is unsigned. In Appendix A of the report, four

individuals are named who "will collect the physiological data during the euthanasia procedure": Preston E. Garraghty, Ph.D. of Vanderbilt University, Jon H. Kaas, Ph.D. of Vanderbilt University, Timothy P. Pons, Ph.D. of NIH, and Peter L. Strick, Ph.D. of the Veterans Administration Hospital.

These individuals were listed in alphabetical order. There is no indication which (if any) of these individuals is the principal investigator. In federal court proceedings on January 12, 1990, NIH attorneys produced a one-page document that they stated contained the names of nine individuals who had written the NIH protocol and sent it to Dr. Raub. They are Robert E. Burke, M.D. (NINCDS, NIH), Michael E. Goldberger, Ph.D. (Medical College of Pennsylvania), Edward G. Jones, M.D., Ph.D. (University of California, Irvine), Jon H. Kaas, Ph.D. (Vanderbilt University), Frederick A. King, Ph.D. (Yerkes Regional Primate Research Center), Mortimer Mishkin, Ph.D. (NIMH), Timothy P. Pons, Ph.D. (NIMH), Peter L. Strick, Ph.D. (Syracuse VA Medical Center/SUNY Syracuse), and William D. Willis, Jr., M.D., Ph.D. (University of Texas Medical Branch, Galveston). Given the protocol's extraordinary brevity and poor quality, it is difficult to believe that these nine signatories actually lent the full benefit of their expertise to writing the protocol.

Among the signatories is Frederick King, who was named in the confidential American Physiological Society memo as being involved in raising funds to execute an agreement among Tulane, the NIH, and representatives of several scientific societies in order to solve the NIH's public relations problem by transferring ownership of the monkeys to Tulane in exchange for private payments. Killing the deafferented monkeys was discussed in the memo as a means of reducing the cost of this arrangement.

In an application to the Institutional Animal Care and Use Committee submitted by Delta Director Peter Gerone on October 20, 1988, Gerone listed himself as the principal investigator. It appears that he assumed this responsibility after the protocol was written. There is no indication that he played any part in drafting the protocol, and he has no relevant expertise. The main responsibility for the application process and for assuring the proper conduct of research rests with the principal investigator. How Gerone assumed this role is unclear.

2. Portions of the text are virtually identical to a report of the panel making recommendations for the monkeys on March 16-18, 1988, entitled "Assessment of and Recommendations for the 'Silver Spring Monkeys.'" In the January 14, 1990 court hearing, NIH attorneys described the "Assessment" report as having been generated by an "independent" panel of experts, who

had decided on the need for euthanasia of some of the monkeys independent of any research consideration. The NIH attorneys used this claim in support of their argument for carrying out the experiment. Nonetheless, it appears that the two documents were not generated independently. The first paragraph of the protocol section entitled "Background of the Scientific Problem" of the NIH proposal reads:

> Damage to the human brain or spinal cord is regarded as irreversible. Nevertheless, it is well documented by clinicians and basic scientists alike that, in the first months after injury, some recovery of function occurs spontaneously. Although this recovery can sometimes be enhanced by efforts at rehabilitation, the results are generally disappointing. One reason that more substantial recovery cannot be induced is that we do not yet understand the mechanisms responsible for the limited improvement that does occur.

In the Delta panel report, the beginning of the first paragraph on page six reads:

> Damage to the human brain and spinal cord has generally been regarded as irreversible. Nevertheless, it is well documented that some recovery of function frequently occurs. While this recovery can sometimes be enhanced by current modes of rehabilitation therapy, the results are generally disappointing. At present, we cannot induce more substantial recovery because of our limited understanding of the neural mechanisms responsible for the slight improvements that do occur.

A comparison of the corresponding second paragraphs of each report reveals more similarities in both structure and language -- similarities beyond those that could be expected in the work of independent writers. The only signatory to both is Raub, who was an "information resource" to the panel and the signatory on letters accompanying the NIH proposal sent to members of Congress. It is not, however, entirely clear which document was generated first.

3. The protocol is undated. This is significant in and of itself, but is also important from the standpoint of the independence of the decision to euthanize the monkeys. Raub's cover letter to members of Congress implies that the protocol was written after the panel decided on euthanasia for two of the monkeys in March, 1988:

> On several occasions we have discussed the fact that all eight of the

> surgically disabled Silver Spring monkeys are likely to require euthanasia eventually. . . . The report on the March site visit to the Delta Regional Primate Research Center. . . . strongly reinforces these expectations. Staff of the Department of Health and Human Services and collaborators therefore have prepared a plan for the euthanasia.

However, the document presented by NIH attorneys in the January 12, 1990 hearing listing nine individuals was dated September 30, 1987, six months before the panel met. The attorneys represented it as a cover letter for the NIH protocol, although it was a loose document in a different typeface and it apparently was not included with the protocol when it was sent to members of Congress or to Delta's Institutional Animal Care and Use Committee.

On January 25, 1990, Raub again stated in a letter to Senator Paul Simon that the protocol was "developed in 1988." The process of deciding whether any of the primates required euthanasia appears to have been intertwined with the desire to conduct the experiment.

4. No site is specified for the research. The experiment was conducted on Billy on January 14, 1990 at Delta. Although the proposal states that the research will occur when "the attending veterinarians at the Delta Primate Center decide that a particular deafferented animal must be euthanised," the proposal does not restrict the experiment to Delta. The four "investigators" mentioned above are described as working at various other institutions; none is listed as a Delta employee. If the research was to be conducted at Delta, it was not specified in which laboratory or under whose supervision that work would be conducted. This information is submitted in all research protocols, for two important reasons: It is critical in determining facilities' suitability for the research in question; it also indicates responsibility for adherence to federal research regulations. Failure to specify the research site is a major omission.

5. The protocol's presentation of the field is deficient. The protocol presents only selected information that does not reflect the depth of current knowledge about the sequelae of neurological damage or of the treatments that are available or under investigation. Properly written research proposals contain a review of relevant scientific literature justifying the proposed research. The NIH protocol contains no mention of *any* specific research in the area in question; it relies solely on vague, undocumented allusions to recent research. The introduction makes a variety of unsupported claims about the animals apparently aimed at lay readers; it bears no resemblance to the introductory comments appropriate to a scientific proposal.

The section entitled "Background of the Scientific Problem" suggests that the current experiment will investigate the rate-limiting variable in neural regeneration. It omits the fact that a number of research teams are conducting research in recovery from brain and nerve damage.[3] It is precisely because regenerative processes are known to occur that numerous researchers have studied them in detail. Selzer[4] has written, "In many cases considerable recovery is seen. Several factors are known to influence the probability and quality of nerve regeneration."

The protocol states that neural regeneration ("sprouting") following spinal cord damage has never before been demonstrated in primates. This is untrue. Bernstein and Bernstein[5] demonstrated sprouting in the spinal cords of rhesus monkeys. The current group of monkeys have severed dorsal roots, and would, therefore, suffer degeneration of axonal processes in the spinal cord. The text of the NIH protocol indicates gross inattention or lack of current knowledge of the research area in question.

6. The protocol uses inappropriate language and unsubstantiated hyperbolic statements in an attempt to build a case for the monkeys' research value. The second paragraph on page two of the protocol presents sweeping statements of conjecture as if they were fact, in an effort to demonstrate that the monkeys in question hold the key to elucidating the mechanisms of recovery from stroke or other neurological injury:

> But pursuing the original [research] plan alone would yield only a small fraction of the information regarding neural plasticity that we now know these animals can provide. That is, the partially deafferented animals have come to represent a scientific resource far beyond that anticipated when Dr. Taub prepared them.

The paragraph then lists reasons why those statements should be considered true. In summary, the reasons are:

a. It is now known that, after brain injury, there can be some functional reorganization of the cortex.

b. Methods (unspecified) for characterizing various neurochemical pathways are becoming available.

c. Techniques (unspecified) now allow a more accurate and thorough study of the changes that occur in the spinal cord after transection of the dorsal root sensory fibers.

These points provide no substantiation for the assertion that the animals in question are "a scientific resource far beyond that anticipated when Dr. Taub prepared them," or that they are even suitable subjects for any meaningful research. There is substantial reason to believe that these animals are not suitable subjects for further research and that the NIH protocol offers no suitable research design.

Moreover, although NIH officials have stated that the experiment is related to stroke, neither they, nor the protocol's author(s) acknowledged the serious problems -- well known to neurologists -- with animal models of stroke and other forms of brain injury. In *Stroke* editorial, Molinari[6] bemoaned that results from animal experiments repeatedly fail to be replicated in human clinical trials. Neff replied:

> The real problem faced by researchers in cerebrovascular disease is that many treatments for stroke have been validated in animal models but then failed in human trials. If the human trials are valid and if the laboratory studies are valid, then the problem must be that the laboratory models are not applicable to human cerebrovascular disease.
>
> This conclusion is not surprising in light of the obvious differences in scale between the human brain and that of rabbits or small primates. . . . The repeated failure of laboratory-proven stroke therapies in humans can be due only to the inapplicability of animal models to human cerebrovascular disease.[7]

Neither of these authors would have attempted to totally discount animal experiments. It is clearly unfounded, however, to hold that animal models of stroke, and particularly this group of monkeys, are nearly certain to lead to rapid and major strides in neurological research or clinical treatments. Another *Stroke* editorial, January, 1990, decried the waste of resources caused by animal experiments in stroke treatment:

> Each time one of these potential treatments is observed to be effective based upon animal research, it propagates numerous further animal and human studies consuming enormous amounts of time and effort to prove that the observation has little or no relevance to human disease or that it may have been an artifact of the animal model itself.[8]

Stroke can be due to many factors, and neural regeneration is one aspect of a complex process. One could make a case that animal experiments are more applicable in certain areas than in others. Nonetheless, no reservations about the applicability to humans of animal experiments in brain function were noted in the protocol.

The protocol's language is highly unusual. Rather than conforming to the norm of specific scientific terminology that unambiguously indicates the place of the proposed research in the relevant field of endeavor, the protocol uses lay terms to dramatize the project's supposed value. The language appears to aim at readers other than scientists. Curiously, at several points in the protocol, technical terms are introduced that would confuse the lay reader but are far too vague to satisfy scientists. For example, "experts in limb pathology," "state-of-the-art immunocytochemical, histochemical, and histological techniques," and "normal control material already in hand" are all used with no further description. These terms provide only a scientific aura without meaningful content. Whether the primary intended readers were the members of Congress to whom the protocol was sent or others is not discernible from the content. The protocol's major deviations from accepted norms suggest that the protocol's intended effect was other than scientific advancement.

7. The proposal' outlined goals and methods are grossly deficient. The proposal specifies three goals, followed by a one-paragraph method section. The goals are vaguely addressed, there is no description of specific hypotheses, and the methods to be used are described in only cursory terms in language aimed at lay readers. All properly written protocols describe the scientific methods in detail. The method section is of interest with regard to the scientific design's adequacy. This design ordinarily includes any examinations or measurements to be made, statistical treatments of data, and the procedures in which animal subjects will be used. The protocol's method section contains only three sentences regarding the euthanasia; there is no mention of the anesthetic agent(s) to be used or the route of administration. This is followed by one brief sentence related to the method to be used in pursuit of the first goal. Two sentences then describe monitoring the animals to avoid pain. A final sentence is devoted to the methods to be used in pursuit of the second and third goals. Although a few more details on methods can be gleaned from the description of the goals, virtually all of the methodologic details are left to the reader's imagination. Each goal and its associated method are discussed below.

a. "To determine the extent of the physiological changes in the somatosensory cortical fields that have resulted from the prolonged deafferentation of the forelimb."

The proposal notes that if the sensory nerves from a given body part, such as a finger or an arm, are severed, the portion of the brain that had previously received input from that body part may begin to receive input from other body areas. The proposal states that it would be useful to know whether the portions of the brain that had served an arm reorganized, after deafferentation of the arm, to receive input from other body parts. The proposal asserts that this research is significant because no researcher has previously investigated reorganization of an area as large as that representing an entire arm, and because a prolonged period of time has elapsed since the experimental injuries.

The proposed method is accorded only one sentence: "During this time the somatosensory cortex will be exposed and a microelectrode used to detect the responses of single neurons to gentle stimulation of the body surface with a camel's-hair brush."

The proposal makes the sweeping prediction that the "euthanasia procedure will not only provide essential information regarding previously unstudied dimensions of neural plasticity following injury, but will also have broad theoretical implications." This is unsupported conjecture presented as a fact.

The protocol further states that "evidence of extensive reorganization in cases of chronic deafferentation would indicate that neural activity is important in maintaining or establishing not just topographic maps but perhaps all forms of sensory representation in the cortex."

Among the protocol's failures is the absence of any rationale that relates the brain mapping to the clinical conditions of stroke and spinal cord injury. The rearrangement of sensory fields is a normal phenomenon that has long been known to occur and would simply be passively observed by the investigators. They are not investigating methods for changing the brain representations, nor are they attempting to alter brain function in motor areas, which are of particular concern in stroke. In stroke, part of the brain is dead; the principal sequelae of concern are motor deficits. While neuropsychologists have long been curious about brain maps, there is no connection between brain mapping and any foreseeable stroke treatments.

There are several deficiencies in the protocol:

i. No hypotheses are stated.

ii. No study design is given. There is no description of what comparisons would be made or what findings would be considered significant.

iii. The methods for measuring neural function are not described. There is no mention as to which cells would be examined, what sort of microelectrode would be used, what measurements would be made, or which body parts would be stimulated in attempts to elicit responses. The type of microelectrode and specifics regarding its use are critical considerations in such an experiment: Some investigators have been concerned that the damage caused by multiple microelectrode penetrations of the cortex may actually modify the cortical representations under study.[9]

iv. Valid and reliable results are not likely to be obtained. In owl monkeys and squirrel monkeys, there is a great deal of variation in the cortical representations of body surfaces from one individual to the next, which may also be true for crab-eating macaques (*Macaca fascicularis*). Evidence suggests that this variation is as great or greater between individuals of the same species as between species.[11,12]

Macaca fascicularis is not the species most commonly used in cortical mapping. Most data in this area come from owl monkeys and squirrel monkeys because their neurological structures facilitate detailed mapping.[11] According to Dr. Taub's 1979 grant application, crab-eating macaques were used because the rhesus monkeys Taub had been using were in short supply.

The variability of cortical representations is likely to be even greater as the brain reorganizes in deafferented subjects. Reorganization is often idiosyncratic. The subsequent experience of the animals further increases this neurological variation.

In cases of high variability, a large sample is required in order to achieve statistical significance. The group of monkeys is small and varied, and continues to dwindle through fatalities. It currently consists of a total of six deafferented *Macaca fascicularis* monkeys and a non-deafferented rhesus female. Of the six, five have a deafferented arm in place and one had his deafferented arm amputated (not by scientific design, but as a remedy for uncontrollable self-inflicted damage). The monkey already experimented on (Billy) was bilaterally deafferented. This small and varied group is far from that expected in standard research.

The word "sample" could be applied to the brain cells measured, rather than the group of animals, but in this case there remains little likelihood of a sufficient sample size. The protocol limits the experiment to a four-hour period prior to killing the animals. The number of measurements of brain cell function that are possible within that time period is relatively small. In court testimony on January 12, 1990, Mortimer Mishkin of the NIMH stated that, at most, 90 to 100 measurements could be made. Brain mapping usually requires extensive sampling, in part because the boundaries between some cortical areas may be poorly defined and overlapping. Selecting a small sample of neurons yields a very coarse result that is difficult to interpret.[9,12]

Variability among animals appears to be due to two factors, genetics and experience, neither of which has been controlled in this group of animals. Since the crab-eating macaques Taub used were captured in the Philippine forest, their genetic backgrounds are entirely unknown. Experiential factors may exert an even more profound effect on the cortical map. Researchers have suggested that the use of the arm may continually modify the cortical representations that the proposal aims to measure. Jenkins and Merzenich[10] report, "In detail, these cortical representations are constantly changing. At least many of these changes must reflect the dominant use history of the animal."

For this group of animals, the use of their arms in the intervening years since their deafferentation has been unstructured, unstandardized, and undocumented, making it highly unlikely that meaningful results can be obtained. As stated in the proposal's introduction, the monkeys did not receive the full schedule of retraining in Taub's original research protocol. The surviving group represents different variants of surgical procedures, as noted above. Moreover, according to veterinary reports, the condition of the deafferented arm differs from one animal to the next. All have had a greater or lesser degree of damage to the deafferented arm, and serious illnesses and fatalities have occurred. X-rays have documented spinal and skeletal changes, which may or may not affect the experience of the animals in ways that could influence the mapping experiment's results. The protocol itself is set to begin when the subjects are so debilitated that euthanasia is required for humane reasons. At that point, serious medical conditions, including possible metabolic and nutritional abnormalities, will be present. None of these effects is accounted for in the protocol. These are highly contaminated research subjects;

In addition, animals whose clinical course has been so poor that euthanasia is required are unlikely to be models for successful recovery. As Raub wrote on October 2, 1985, "We have no research protocols, either ongoing or planned, for which these animals are appropriate."

v. There are no control animals. Taub's surviving control monkeys have been moved to the San Diego Zoo and are in group housing. These differences in setting, along with the lack of control over the experiences of the animals in both groups for the past eight years, would be expected to lead to significant differences in the brain functions to be measured. The protocol's descriptions of the use of control samples reflect little understanding of the use of controls in scientific study.

vi. Confounding effects of anesthesia, age, illness, and medical treatments are neglected in the proposal. Some researchers[13,14] have found significant effects of anesthetic agents on cortical mapping experiments; others[15] have not. The failure to describe the anesthetic agent intended for use and to address the issue of potential artifact introduced thereby is a serious omission. In addition, age affects the capacity for cortical reorganization in some species.[16]

vii. A key variable in Taub's work -- the behavioral assessment describing the capacity of the animals to use their deafferented limbs -- was abandoned several years ago. Experience is a key element in brain somatotopographic representations. Without this information, there is no basis on which to judge the significance of brain restructuring, even if it could be accurately measured, and no applicability of this experiment to the rehabilitation of nerve injuries. NIH spokespersons have stated that one of the experiment's goals is to facilitate rehabilitation of victims of spinal cord injury and stroke, yet no part of the experiment relates to treatment or rehabilitation. The proposal's claim of clinical significance ("potentially of great significance for alleviating suffering and advancing human health") this would be grandiose even if the protocol were more carefully constructed and properly written. Cortical mapping is "basic research," not clinical research. The finding that intact body parts make connections with portions of the brain that previously represented deafferented body parts is not directly related to the functional recovery of the deafferented body part. There is no relationship to current or proposed clinical treatments. The proposal asserts that this research will aid in the development of "strategies aimed at promoting functional recovery from nerve injury," but provides no rationale as to why this might be an expected outcome. The experiences of the animals, who for the past eight years have been confined to small individual enclosures with no rehabilitative interventions, no exercise or even freedom of movement, and no normal social interactions, are dramatically different from the rehabilitative efforts that would normally follow neurological injury in humans.

There is no evident basis for the contention that this group of animals is appropriate to research in this area. There has been essentially no control and considerable artifact in the intervening years. The sample is so small, varied, and uncontrolled that achieving statistically significant results is extremely unlikely.

b. "To identify the immunocytochemical changes in cortex or thalamus that might underlie the physiological changes."

The protocol states that, when portions of the brain change their organization (for example, to receive input from a new body part), these changes in brain organization may relate to changes in the quantities of neurotransmitters present in those parts of the brain. It then states that the quantity of neurotransmitters present may be influenced by activity in the body parts in question. Speculations then follow, suggesting that information from this study could help in "phantom limb pain" or recovery of function following deafferentation.

The protocol then proposes, with no supporting rationale, the measurement of cytochrome oxidase, GABA, glutamate, Substance P, CAM-II, protein kinase C, C-fos, and CAT-301. The protocol states that these measurements will be used to see "whether changes in quantities of neurotransmitters in the cortex are due to changes in metabolism or neurotransmitters in the thalamus." They will also be used to search for changes in other unspecified parts of the cortex.

As with the first goal, no model or hypothesis is specified, and there is no experimental design. The techniques by which samples will be obtained, how assays will be done, how the results will be analyzed, and what degrees of differences in measurements would achieve statistical significance are not specified. Anesthetic effects are not discussed.

The text suggests that immunocytochemical techniques would be used for the assays noted above. Although no specific fixative is noted in the protocol, the IACUC application calls for the use of glutaraldehyde. This chemical would cause great distortion of the antigenic proteins, precluding most of the intended measurements. Sternberger[17] has described two major problems with the fixative:

> Glutaraldehyde seems to destroy, in most instances, detectability of antigen by immunofluorescence. . . . Glutaraldehyde, by virtue of its cross-linking qualities, hardens tissues so much that it prevents its own penetration, whether in perfusion or immersion fixations.

Although no hypotheses are stated, three are implied and can be separated for discussion purposes:

i. Chemical levels in deafferented sections of the brain differ from levels on the contralateral side.

The protocol calls for separate measurements of eight chemicals in five monkeys, assuming that only unilaterally deafferented monkeys with arms in place are used. Each subject provides his own control. This requires a minimum of 40 comparisons. If the significance level is set at .05, then by chance alone results would appear significant in two of the 40 comparisons. The investigators are particularly vulnerable to this error given that there is no prediction as to the expected results; they are, in essence, "fishing." To minimize this source of error, a stricter criterion for statistical significance (e.g., .01) is required. With the small sample, as discussed above, and a strict criterion for significance, achieving significant results will be difficult.

A further flaw is the absence of any discussion of the differences that may normally be expected between the two cerebral hemispheres of *Macaca fascicularis*.

ii. Brain chemical levels in experimental subjects are outside the range for normal subjects.

If a difference is found between the experimental monkeys and "normals," there is no way to attribute the cause of the difference. The protocol indicates that measurements will be compared between the deafferented monkeys and unspecified "normal control material already in hand." The word "control" does not refer simply to normal tissue or normal individuals. "Control" refers to a comparison sample that has undergone precisely the same treatments as the experimental group, with the exception of the experimental variable in question. For the "material already in hand" to act as a control, it would have to have come from monkeys who had experienced the same treatment, other than the experimental manipulations, and the same subsequent experience as the animals who had undergone the experimental procedures. Age, medical conditions and all other factors that could influence results should also be essentially the same. There are no monkeys who meet these criteria, particularly since very few of Taub's original control monkeys are still alive, and all of these are in an entirely different setting from Delta and have long deviated from the procedures Taub had planned.

The protocol calls for taking samples in highly unusual circumstances. The samples would be taken from monkeys who have experienced the prolonged stress of years of isolation caging, illness so severe that euthanasia is necessary, and a final four hours of anesthesia. All of these factors can be expected to affect brain chemical levels. There is no mention as to whether control animals would have undergone similar treatment, nor is it likely that any such animals are available.

iii. There is a relationship between brain chemical levels and the brain representation of body parts.

The protocol seeks "correlations between functional and structural maps for a wide variety of neurochemical factors." The word correlation appears to be used improperly, since it is not possible to calculate a correlation between a linear variable, such as a chemical level, and a structural map.

In summary, gross methodologic problems are apparent for all three implied hypotheses. Without a carefully planned method for comparing results of sufficient numbers of subjects in experimental and control groups who are comparable on relevant variables, measurements are not meaningful.

The text makes two references to anatomical measurements in the cortex and thalamus, once in the title "Anatomy and Cytochemistry of the Somatosensory Cortex and Thalamus" and once in a text sentence: "It should be pointed out that the major value of these anatomical and chemical studies will derive from a comparison with functional data." There is, however, no mention whatsoever of any anatomical examination of the cortex or thalamus in the description of the goals or methods, or anywhere else in the protocol; it appears to have simply been overlooked. In spite of Raub's contention that "This plan is drawn carefully," it appears that the proposal was hastily conceived and written.

There is no reason to believe that the protocol can in any way assist in the two clinical problems noted, nor is there any basis for this speculation in the protocol. The anonymous author did not distinguish between phantom limb pain and phantom limb syndrome, and has not attempted to review or even comment on the literature on either condition that might relate to the protocol.

c. "To look for evidence of 'sprouting' in the spinal cord as originally intended by Dr. Taub, and to determine whether anatomical and cytochemical changes at this level of the system are correlated with reorganizational changes at higher levels."

The protocol states that when afferent nerves of cats or rats are damaged, the remaining intact nerves may "sprout" new connections that will provide a degree of compensation. It states that electron microscopic examination of the spinal cord will assess the presence of "sprouting" in the monkeys. In addition, the biochemical assays which were alluded to above for the cortex will also be applied to samples of the brain stem and spinal cord, and the monkeys' forelimbs will be examined "by experts in limb pathology." The method of tissue fixation is described in the following terms: "the monkey will be perfused with normal saline followed by a dilute aldehyde fixative." The examinations will use "state-of-the-art immunocytochemical, histochemical, and histological techniques."

As noted above, the protocol states that neural regeneration following spinal cord damage has never before been demonstrated in primates. Bernstein and Bernstein,[5] however, published a detailed experiment demonstrating sprouting in the spinal cords of rhesus monkeys.

As in the discussion of the first two goals, there is a marked lack of specificity of the research design and methods. There is no indication as to which parts of the brain stem and spinal cord will be sampled. The "experts in limb pathology," the methods they would use, and what they might be looking for all remain unidentified. Previously discussed concerns regarding the absence of controls apply here as well.

The terms "dilute aldehyde fixative" are not sufficiently specific. Formaldehyde is useful for preparing tissues for examination by light microscopy, but it is inappropriate for electronic microscopy. Glutaraldehyde or a glutaraldehyde/para-formaldehyde solution would be more appropriate for that application but would be inappropriate for the immunocytochemical measures, as noted above. According to the IACUC application submitted by Gerone, glutaraldehyde was to be used.

It appears that the fixative is intended to act as the killing agent. Failure to specify the agent is gross omission. This issue would be of interest to an Institutional Animal Care and Use Committee. It is possible that the saline infusion would wash out certain anesthetics and that, just before death, the aldehyde fixative would be infused into animals no longer properly anesthetized. The lack of specificity in this area prevents the reader from rendering an informed judgment. As is true of the remainder of the protocol, the description's vagueness represents a serious deviation from scientific norms.

No details at all are provided on the methods of tissue examination, how they fit into a research design, how the results will be analyzed, or what will be regarded as a significant finding. Synapses resulting from sprouting can be analyzed in a variety of ways: their number, density, and type; the number of synaptic contacts made by each terminal; the transmitters they contain; etc. The mention of "state-of-the-art immunocytochemical, histochemical, and histological techniques" provides the reader with no evidence that the proposal's author understood which methods would be appropriate for such a study. Such wording is entirely inappropriate for a scientific document.

It must also be noted that the protocol aims to accomplish its task in "no more than four hours." A typical mapping procedure requires several hundred microelectrode penetrations and measurements[11] and takes many hours to complete. The four-hour time limitation, which is difficult to reconcile with the proposed goals, appears to derive from public relations concerns.

The problems with this proposal go beyond its scanty presentation. There is little, if any, scientific basis for using this unusual group of monkeys in this area of research. The grandiose claims that are made are not in keeping with reasonable goals of scientific endeavor.

8. No list of references is appended to the protocol. This is highly improper, as it prevents the reader from verifying the statements in the protocol or seeking additional information.

Critique of Protocol: Administrative Procedures

On or about July 1, 1988, the NIH protocol was sent to Congressmen Robert K. Dornan and Robert Smith, along with a two-page cover letter signed by William F. Raub, then NIH Deputy Director. On August 30, 1988, it was sent to Congressman Charlie Rose. The process by which this plan was submitted is unclear. However, it appears to have deviated markedly from normal procedures required for proposals for federally funded research:

1. There is no evidence that any competitive grant applications were solicited from potential investigators. Raub had, in fact, expressed the NIH's unequivocal lack of interest in this research area in his letter to Dr. Vasapoli (cited above).

2. There is no evidence that the research area in question had been evaluated as to its priority before the proposal's appearance.

3. The Institutional Animal Care and Use Committee (IACUC) should not have been asked to approve the protocol in its present format. The protocol was described by NIH 12, 1990, as a preliminary protocol. The list of presumed authors also described it as preliminary. It is highly improper for an IACUC to approve a project without being presented detailed descriptions of the procedures that animals will undergo and a rationale for the number of animals used and the species chosen. Given that Peter Gerone was both the listed principal investigator and the Delta Center's director, it appears that the Delta IACUC's capacity to render objective judgement was compromised.

Raub clearly intended the NIH protocol to stand on its own; he described it as a finalized document. Moreover, Raub planned for its implementation with no further review. The NIH plan was not offered to the Congressmen as a draft proposal or a summary of another, more comprehensive, document. The cover letter does not state that details will follow, nor is there any suggestion in the proposal or the cover letter that a process of applying for appropriate approvals had begun. Nowhere is there any suggestion that a more detailed protocol is available for review. Raub's cover letter described the proposal as a plan which "is drawn carefully." It was represented as a plan that was to lead directly to the implementation of the research protocol described therein.

In a letter to Congressman Smith on October 13, 1988, Raub unequivocally stated his intention to immediately implement the provisions of the NIH protocol:

> With respect to the most seriously disabled monkeys, we have deferred the euthanasia decision since July at your and Mr. Dornan's request. However, further delay no longer is tenable. . . . On your visit to the Delta Center in late August, you and I discussed the proposed euthanasia protocol in detail. I am grateful to you for the time you invested to understand why the experimentally disabled monkeys are of unique importance to the rehabilitation of handicapped human beings. My colleagues and I plan to proceed in accord with my July 1 letter and attachments, and my subsequent discussions with you, Mr. Dornan, and your staff members. I hope you recognize that the DHHS cannot do otherwise and still honor its mission and responsibilities.

The proposed protocol is not simply a continuation of the original experiments in progress at the time the animals were originally seized; it is a materially different project for which a new approval process is required. Raub's letters to Congressmen Dornan and Smith clearly show that he intended them to believe that the plan had been carefully written and properly proposed, and that he intended to proceed. On January 14, 1990, Gerone and other investigators did so.

Conclusions

The protocol is markedly deficient in many areas. Its format and content are grossly deviant from the norms commonly accepted for scientific research. The research protocol is incomplete, poorly written, and unlikely to achieve meaningful or useful results. The frequent use of inappropriate language and extravagant claims suggests that its intent was to create an impression for lay readers rather than scientists.

This case's history shows that experiments on this group of animals have been advanced for reasons unrelated to science. James Wyngaarden described the Silver Spring Monkeys case as the most enervating part of his tenure as NIH Director. Along with his assistant William Raub, Wyngaarden played an active role in negotiations with Congress and scientific organizations on the case. Numerous scientific organizations have joined the NIH's efforts to advance various experiments on the animals, not for their scientific value, but explicitly in order to prevail in litigation or public controversies. Likewise, the NIH protocol advanced by Raub in 1988 appears to be motivated by reasons other than the advancement of scientific knowledge.

Evidence suggests that the proposal was offered with four possible aims in mind, none of which relate to scientific advancement in the area in question, but all of which assist the NIH in keeping the animals out of the activists' custody and help solve what NIH officials viewed as a major public relations problem:

1. To kill the monkeys. NIH and Delta officials have attempted to make a case for euthanasia based on poorly supported rationales. The research proposal appears to be intended to give added reason for disposing of the animals and, thus, of the possibility of setting any precedent perceived as contrary to the NIH's interests.

Killing the animals would also allow the NIH to rid itself of a longstanding public relations problem. A document from the American Physiological Society specifically calculates how killing the deafferented animals would save money for several professional societies in a plan to free the NIH from its embarrassing role in the case.

2. To indicate to Congress and the courts that the NIH has an important research interest in the animals that justifies their staying at a federal facility, rather than a sanctuary approved by animal protection groups.

3. To justify the continued diversion of NIH resources to litigation or other expenses in the case.

4. To satisfy the curiosity of the experimental neuropsychologists regarding the monkeys' brain function (even though any findings would be compromised by confounding variables and absence of controls).

Review of the NIH protocol and other aspects of this case indicates that there is a willingness on the part of NIH and Delta officials to discard scientific rigor and integrity for the sake of financial and political expediencies. Representatives of several large scientific organizations have privately indicated their willingness to assert the value of research on these animals in order to further the aim of defeating what they perceive as a threat to their own and their organizations' interests.

The use of the plan by Raub and others shows repeated misrepresentations, deception in communications with members of Congress and the courts, and abuse of the scientific process to further other aims.

A full and objective investigation of the circumstances surrounding this case is essential to restoring confidence in the capacity of NIH administrators to make proper decisions concerning the conduct of research and to enforce animal welfare laws. Such an investigation should consider, among the many other indications of misconduct:

The process by which the proposal was developed.

The persistent advocacy activity of Raub and others in this case.

The apparent compromise of scientific judgment that led Raub to repeatedly state to members of Congress and federal judges that the protocol was "carefully" drawn.

The failure to adhere to repeated promises not to conduct invasive experiments on the animals.

The process by which a principal investigator with no expertise in the relevant research area was assigned.

The process by which the protocol (which omitted important details regarding an extended invasive procedure) was approved by the Institutional Animal Care and Use Committee at the institution of which the principal investigator was the director.

The inappropriate attempts to elicit determinations for euthanasia of the animals.

The secret agreement between Tulane University, the NIH, and scientific societies regarding the monkeys and the pressure that agreement may have exerted on the euthanasia decisions.

The grossly deviant process by which the NIH proposal was advanced warrants thorough investigation. Impropriety appears to be well-entrenched in numerous scientific organizations and at the highest levels of the NIH. Robert Windom sent the protocol to Congressman Charlie Rose on August 30, 1988, and, in an accompanying letter, attempted to convince the Congressman that his objections to it were unfounded. Secretary Louis Sullivan wrote to Louisiana Governor Buddy Roemer on May 24, 1989:

> Although we have kept an open mind toward the possibility of relocating a few of the monkeys, we have no intention of entering into any agreement that . . . precludes carrying out the appropriate physiological, histochemical, and histopathological determinations at the time when humane considerations dictate euthanasia.

A full and impartial investigation is urgently needed. There is every reason to believe that research funds, personnel, and materials are easily diverted to non-research purposes, and that truth and objectivity currently have low priority in much federally funded research.

References

1. Gerone PJ: The right to animal research. *Animal Care Matters*, National Institutes of Health, August 1989.
2. Sweet WH: Deafferentation pain in man. *Appl Neurophysiol* 1988;51:117-127.
3. Waxman SG: Functional recovery in diseases of the nervous system. *Adv Neurol* 1988;47:1-7.

4. Selzer ME: Nerve regeneration. *Sem Neurol* 1987;7:88-96.
5. Bernstein ME, Bernstein JJ: Regeneration of axons and synaptic complex formation rostral to the site of hemisection in the spinal cord of the monkey. *Internat J Neurosci* 1973;5:15-26.
6. Molinari GF: Why model strokes? *Stroke* 1988;19:1195-1197.
7. Neff S: Clinical relevance of stroke models. *Stroke* 1989;20:699-700.
8. Wiebers DO, Adams HP, Whisnant JP: Animal models of stroke: Are they relevant to human disease? *Stroke* 1990;21:1-3.
9. Merzenich MM, Kaas JH, Wall JT, Sur M, Nelson RJ, Felleman DJ: Progression of change following median nerve section in the cortical representation of the hand in areas 3b and 1 in adult owl and squirrel monkeys. *Neuroscience* 1983;10:639-665.
10. Merzenich MM, Nelson RJ, Kaas JH, et al: Variability in hand surface representations in areas 3b and 1 in adult owl and squirrel monkeys. *J Compar Neurol* 1987;258:281-296.
11. Jenkins WM, Merzenich, MM: Reorganization of neocortical representations after brain injury: A neurophysiological model of the bases of recovery from stroke. *Prog Brain Res* 1987;71:249-266.
12. Robinson CJ: Somatotopographic organization in the second somatosensory area of *M. fascicularis*. *J Comp Neurol* 1980;192:43-67.
13. Duncan GH, Dreyer DA, McKenna TM, Whitsel BL: Dose- and time-dependent effects of ketamine on SI neurons with cutaneous receptive fields. *J Neurophysiol* 1982;47:677-699.
14. McKenna TM, Whitsel BL, Dreyer DA: Anterior parietal cortical topographic organization in macaque monkey: Re-evaluation. *J Neurophysiol* 1982;48:289-318.
15. Stryker MP, Jenkins WM, Merzenich MM: Anesthetic state does not affect the map of the hand representation within area 3b somatosensory cortex in owl monkey. *J Compar Neurol* 1987;258:297-303.
16. McKinley PA, Jenkins WM, Smith JL, Merzenich MM: Age-dependent capacity for somatosensory cortex reorganization in chronic spinal cats. *Brain Res* 1987;428:136-139.
17. Sternberger LA: *Immunocytochemistry, 3rd Ed*. New York, John Wiley & Sons, 1986.
human disease? *Stroke* 1990;21:1-3.

Evaluation of Bone Graft Research

Neal D. Barnard, M.D.

The Physicians Committee for Responsible has received the expert opinions of several orthopedic surgeons and pathologists regarding the protocols for proposed bone-replacement research on greyhound dogs at the Letterman Army Institute of Research. A thorough evaluation of the project, however, will require more complete information about the experiments. The following is a preliminary analysis, based on the materials we have received to date.

Background

Bone grafting has been an active field in orthopedic research for at least 65 years. Three basic types of bone grafts exists: autografts, in which bone is taken from one part of the patient's body and utilized at another site; allografts which generally involve bone obtained from bone banks; and synthetic grafts.

A variety of synthetic materials have been tested for use in grafting. The most successful to date appears to be coralline hydroxyapatite, a substance manufactured by Interpore International of Irvine, California. This substance, which is produced from the calcium carbonate skeletal structure of reef-building sea corals, has been used as a bone replacement in animal and human studies since 1978 and has received pre-market approval from the Food and Drug Administration (FDA).

Synthetic grafts have limitations. Chief among these is the patient's immunologic response to a foreign substance and the possibility of infection. (Since synthetic materials are not vascularized, it is difficult to deliver antibiotics to the site of the infection.) Oral surgeons once used synthetic bone grafts, but later they all but abandoned the practice due to high infection rates.[1] Potential toxicity and carcinogenicity of synthetic compounds are also concerns.

Justification for the Study

In order to evaluate the need for the proposed study properly, it is necessary to have more information about the 3M synthetic that the Letterman researchers intend to investigate. The protocols indicate that the synthetic has exhibited osteoinductive properties, implying that some testing has been done. Have toxicity and efficacy studies been conducted by the manufacturer? It would be foolish to proceed with large-scale, expensive studies on dogs if the material in question is likely to be toxic to humans. Is there reason to believe that the substance will have advantages over coralline hydroxyapatite, for which substantial data exist?

The Experimental Model

While the canine model has been used extensively in orthopedic research, its clinical relevance is less than clear. For example, Pierre M. Galleti, professor of medical science and head of the graduate program in artificial organs and biomaterials at Brown University, described the inadequacies of animal models in this type of research. In 1988, he wrote:

> Research using animals simply will not suffice ... The replacement of wrists, knees, hips and finger joints generally poses complex engineering problems because of the heavy mechanical loads involved and the range of motion required. Since there is no generally accepted large-animal model for most of the bones and joints that orthopedic devices are designed to replace, clinical evaluation in humans is the most significant test. Finally, humans live much longer than most animals. For prostheses that are intended to last a lifetime, animal studies are inadequate.[2]

The criticism is relevant to bone graft research as well, because many of the same parameters -- compatibility, durability, toxicity -- are involved.

While the research protocol states that other animal models are inappropriate because of anatomical and biomechanical differences, it does not explain why the dog is an appropriate model for this kind of study. It may be that the dog is better than other animal models, but it does not necessarily mean that the dog model is adequate for clinically applicable investigations in bone replacement.

In addition, the use of former race dogs may introduce complicating variables to the experiment. It is known that these dogs commonly sustain stress fractures, ligament damage and other injuries, and the effect of these factors on the ultimate success of the bone grafts is unknown and unaccounted for in these protocols.

Finally, the protocols state that the fibula has been the typical model for bone repair in the dog. Why is it necessary to establish a new model, using the femur as the site for bone grafting? The protocol states that the femur is more highly vascularized, but it does not explain why this is a better model than the fibula, for which there is extensive research experience. One wonders whether the 3M synthetic has already been tested unsuccessfully in the fibula.

Model for Battlefield Injury

The goal of the experiments is to explore alternative methods of fracture treatment to expedite the healing of long bone injuries suffered in combat. Surgical defects will be created in the dogs without significant injury to surrounding nerves and blood vessels, and without loss of surrounding tissue. Yet, a critical element of bone healing is the viability of the soft tissues, particularly the blood vessels, around the injury site. Bone fractures always damage these tissues, and the damage is particularly severe in military wounds. This experimental protocol, which carefully avoids soft tissue damage, is fundamentally different from any kind of human traumatic bone fracture. It is ironic that the military is funding this research, because the model least applies to military-type orthopedic injuries.

The protocol states that "the vast majority of these soldiers have fractures which are open, comminuted and contaminated." Indeed, battlefield wounds are particularly susceptible to infection. Yet the surgical defect is created under sterile conditions, thus eliminating the possibility of infections. Furthermore, as stated before, the problem of infection is a serious one for synthetic bone replacement. The use of synthetic grafts for the type of wounds sustained by soldiers in combat, is likely to be very problematic, at best.

Costs

The proposed study, if completed, would involve as many as 112 retired greyhound race dogs. According to the protocols, the cost of purchasing these dogs would be $41,000 and housing them for the duration of the experiment would cost as much at $48,000. The costs of other supplies and salaries for personnel, combined with the $89,000 for purchase and housing of the dogs, make this experiment an expensive endeavor. There are also legitimate humane concerns. After creating painful skeletal defects, the protocols state that analgesics and sedatives will be provided "as needed." However, no criteria for such decisions are mentioned. The way in which the researchers intend to prevent the dogs from harming the surgical site is unclear.

Summary

The fracture-repair experiments proposed by researchers at the Letterman Army Institute of Research are costly, both in terms of tax dollars and animal suffering. The Army's reluctance to release the name of the compound to be investigated is puzzling in light of the fact that the material is already patented. Clearly, information about the compound's toxicity and potential for success is necessary before the experiments proceed. We presume that relevant information addressing these concerns exists, but it is not provided in the research protocols. Furthermore, information about the researchers' backgrounds and experience in the field of bone replacement research and a bibliography of papers which describe the strengths and weaknesses of existing animal models are necessary for a thorough evaluation of this proposal. Such documentation would be provided routinely in a grant application to the National Institute of Health.

Based on the information available to us, the proposed model for bone replacement study appears scientifically flawed and not worthy of funding. Should more information become available, we will most certainly consult our orthopedic surgeons and pathologists for a more complete evaluation.

References

1. Orthopedic and Rehabilitation Devices Panel of the FDA: Transcript of a meeting. June 6, 1989.

2. Galletti PM: Artificial organs: Learning to live with risk. *Technology Review* Nov/Dec 1988, pp 35-40.

Book Reviews

C.F.M. Hendriksen: *Laboratory Animals in Vaccine Production and Control: Replacement, Reduction and Refinement.*

Kluwer Academic Publishers, Boston, 1988, 158pp., $49.50.

This book reviews the current use and misuse of animals in human and animal vaccination. Hendriksen provides detailed analysis of current methods of vaccine development and safety-testing. He points out where and how animal use could readily be eliminated or reduced. For example, if uniform guidelines replaced the individual and haphazard methods of testing and quality control currently used by different nations and manufacturers, a substantial decrease in animal use would immediately occur.

For the most part, Hendriksen focuses on tests that may be refined or abandoned in order to reduce animal use. The goal of seeking alternatives is a worthy one. The word "alternatives," however, may falsely suggest that the choice is among protocols of equal scientific validity. Importantly, Hendriksen notes that the animal tests can be misleading and that developing non-animal methodologies is, therefore, desirable not only from an animal protection standpoint, but also in the interest of improved scientific reliability. The cholera vaccine, for example, tested safe and effective in animal models but not in humans.

Although Hendriksen notes several examples of dangerously misleading results from animal tests, he goes to considerable lengths to assure the reader that he generally supports animal experimentation as a scientifically legitimate, although ethically questionable, activity. He makes the undemonstrated claim, "It cannot be denied that a large part of modern health care is based on knowledge acquired through experiments on live animals."

Hendriksen does provide some evidence that animal research has contributed to our understanding of infectious diseases. For example, animals have served as "living test tubes" to harbor infectious agents, thereby permitting study of the infectious organisms themselves. The role of animal research in this regard, however, has decreased considerably since the early 20th century, because *in vitro* cultures tend to be much more efficient, inexpensive, and controllable than *in vivo* preparations. Hendriksen also points out that animals have, by Koch's postulates, "proved" the virulence of infectious organisms. Often, however, Koch's postulates fail to serve: many organisms that produce disease in humans are non-pathogenic in other species.

Overall, Hendriksen does not give sufficient credit to the role of clinical investigation. He fails, for example, to mention Lady Montague's introduction of Jenner's cowpox/small pox vaccination into Western society -- an event that initiated the modern era of vaccination. Although I take issue with Hendriksen's broad endorsement of animal research as a scientifically valuable enterprise, his survey of strategies to reduce animal use in vaccine production and control is informative and quite comprehensive.

Ron Allison, M.D.

Gill Langley (Ed.): *Animal Experimentation: The Consensus Changes.*

Routledge, Chapman and Hall, New York, 1989, 268 pp., $15.95 pap.

Dr. Gill Langley has edited a valuable book that presents a broad range of viewpoints on different aspects of the animal research controversy. Mary Midgley's opening essay ("Are you an animal?") is itself worth the book's price. Midgley expands on some of her earlier essays to address our confused notions about the nature of animals and our relationship to the nonhuman animal world. Her critique of behaviorist psychology is also illuminating.

In a concise critique, Dr. Erik Millstone points out the limitations of current animal tests in toxicology. His recommendations, however, are disappointing. He suggests, for example, that improvements in the animal tests will increase their value. While this may be true to some extent, the animal tests will always be compromised by inter-species differences in anatomy and physiology. Computer models and *in vitro* techniques have much more potential for further refinement and improved reliability. Millstone should have explored the potential of newer non-animal methodologies.

Clive Hollands identifies several types of research that he finds "trivial and questionable." In support of his view, he offers such well-known examples as the Draize test, the LD50 test, and Dr. Edward Taub's experiments at the Institute for Behavioral Research. Hollands also provides examples likely to be new to many familiar with the animal research debate.

Several authors provide needed updates on general topics. Dr. Martin

Stephens discusses alternatives to animal experiments. He argues that wider use of these research methodologies should ultimately improve the quality of science. Stephens stresses the importance of non-animal research in past scientific achievements. Rose and Adams contribute an interesting essay on the scientific evidence for pain and suffering in nonhuman animals. They draw on anatomical, biochemical, and behavioral data to make inferences about animals' subjective experiences.

Several essays deal with animal protection legislation. Holly Hazard and Dr. Judith Hampson provide overviews of American and European initiatives. Dr. David Morton stresses the role of the Animals (Scientific Procedures) Act of 1986 in protecting experimental animals. While he expresses optimism regarding this legislation's impact, he acknowledges that researchers' degree of compliance will largely be unmonitored by any outside agency. Animal protectionists have long noted researchers' failure to self-monitor. I am, therefore, less optimistic than Morton. I also take issue with Morton's underlying premise that good animal welfare ensures good science. If the model is invalid, the results will be irrelevant, whether or not the animals are housed in sanitary, low-stress environments.

In other essays written on the topic, Dr. Tom Regan opposes vivisection on animal rights grounds. The basis of Regan's moral argument is that the sentience of other animals should preclude their use as mere tools intended to serve human ends. Dr. Robert Sharpe's paper, which challenges animal models' scientific validity, is based on his recently published book *The Cruel Deception*. Sharpe argues that the diversion of scarce research funds to animal experimentation and such experimentation's dearth of meaningful results outweigh any past benefits animal research may have provided.

Dr. Gill Langley addresses issues not covered by the other contributors, including the use of animals in education and the duplicity of the campaign to defend animal research. Arrogance and elitism, she maintains, account for the animal research community's refusal to seriously address concerns raised by the public and by scientific colleagues. She argues that this entrenchment at least partly reflects insensitivity to animal protection concerns. This insensitivity, in turn, partly derives from an educational system that intentionally desensitizes young scientists to animal suffering. While she provides few new data, her essay is concise and forceful.

This collection of well-written and thoughtful essays is clearly designed to help bridge the wide gap between the animal protection movement and the animal research community. Historically, researchers have enjoyed considerable autonomy. Whether, inspired by publications like this book, they will endorse reform remains to be seen. I have my doubts, given the animal research community's current strategy of defending nearly every project as both humane and vitally essential for human well-being. A growing segment of the public, however, is challenging the methods of animal research on scientific and/or ethical grounds. In these austere times, growing discontent with the animal research community may force it to re-think its presently intransigent position.

Kathryn Hahner, Ph.D.

Alan M Goldberg (Ed.): *In Vitro Toxicology: New Directions.*

Mary Ann Liebert, New York, 1989, 350 pp., $130.

In Vitro Toxicology: New Directions is the seventh volume in the Alternative Methods in Toxicology Series. This collection of papers from the Center for Alternatives to Animal Testing's 1989 symposium examines *in vitro* techniques for product discovery, product development, and toxicology.

The first part, comprised of papers from the oral presentations, addresses product development, insulin assays, neurotoxicity, and immunotoxicity. O. Hurko's paper "Permanent differentiated cell lines from human biopsy material" describes a particularly exciting new method, in which a zinc-containing culture medium allows unlimited replication of human muscle cells. When the zinc is removed, the cells revert to their terminally differentiated state. While Hurko admits that this system needs refinement, it may eventually be used to grow a small number of diseased human cells into a much larger quantity of cells, thereby permitting a wide range of studies.

The second part, derived from the poster presentations, covers a wide range of subjects, including *in vitro* methods for studying dermal, hepatic, ocular, reproductive, developmental, and immunotoxicity. As a research biologist/dermatologist, I took a special interest in papers dealing with dermal toxicity. In fact, our own laboratory has adopted the system described by Naughton et al. in their paper "A physiologic skin model for *in vitro* toxicity studies." Naughton et al. report growth of human fibroblasts cultured on a pretreated nylon mesh. They propose seeding human epithelial cells onto the fibroblasts and then performing dermal toxicity tests on these cells. In our laboratory, we have replaced animal skin with this system to study collagen, a major protein constituent of the dermis. So far, the results have been highly encouraging. We are now beginning to use this cell culture system to study a variety of collagen-related skin diseases in humans.

This volume offers much interesting and valuable information. Many of the *in vitro* systems are rather crude and simplistic, but they provide a foundation on which to base more sophisticated methods. As concern about the scientific reliability and morality of traditional animal tests grows, this ongoing series should assist the development of non-animal tests.

Paul Contard, Ph.D., M.D.

Bernard E. Rollin, *The Unheeded Cry: Animal Consciousness, Animal Pain and Science*

Oxford University Press, New York, 1989, 308 pp., $29.95.

Common sense notions, Bernard Rollin points out in *The Unheeded Cry*, are not always correct. For example, the law that two objects dropped from the same height will fall at the same speed, regardless of their mass (and discounting air resistance), defies most people's intuitions. In Rollin's view, physics, operating through the application of methodical measuring techniques, is an objective science that leads to increasingly accurate understanding of natural phenomena.

On the other hand, denial of the common sense notion that nonhuman animals possess consciousness and feel pain has not improved our understanding of human or nonhuman psychology. Instead, behaviorism has inflicted great suffering on nonhuman animals while failing to increase understanding.

In developing his case for nonhuman consciousness, Rollin demonstrates that the denial of such consciousness by modern psychologists did not arise because previous theories were proven wrong. Rather, behaviorism arose *de novo* because psychologists wanted to be seen as "hard" scientists who could describe behavior in objective terms. Shunning such supposedly anthropomorphic and subjective words as *fear* and *anxiety*, psychologists who shocked a dog into immobility reported instead that the dog *urinated*, *defecated*, *trembled*, or *whimpered*.

With the behaviorist approach, researchers could not only wear the appearance of greater objectivity but also ignore any suffering they inflicted. In dismissing the consideration of suffering, however, animal researchers overlook an important variable -- the effect of laboratory stress on nonhuman animals. Ironically, experiments with nonhuman animals have shown that the laboratory environment alone causes changes in behavior, physiology, and immunology -- negating the researcher's claims of accuracy and validity.

The Unheeded Cry is packed with information, yet always remains readable. Rollin illustrates his points with personal anecdotes, as well as a detailed review of the literature. While most of the book deals with psychology research, Rollin also demonstrates how behaviorism influences practices in biological research and in confinement rearing of animals for food production.

Unfortunately, Rollin's authority is somewhat undermined by sexist and speciesist language. In places, Rollin does use "he or she" to refer to people in general; more often, however, he resorts to the generic "he." Similarly, Rollin frequently refers to a nonhuman individual as "he" or "she," but he also falls into the use of "it" or "thing." Since the book's goal is to show that nonhuman animals possess consciousness and are therefore above the level of mere things, Rollin's language is inconsistent with his aims.

In the end, Rollin builds a compelling case for rejecting the behaviorist approach and being guided by the overwhelming evidence -- and most people's intuitive recognition -- that nonhuman animals think and feel. Unfortunately, he is too optimistic in his conclusion that behaviorism in science, particularly in psychology, has already been abandoned.

Eric Dunayer, V.M.D.

Medical Research Modernization Committee

The MRMC is comprised of health care professionals who lend their training, experience, and expertise to evaluate the medical and/or scientific merit of research modalities in order to identify archaic methods and to promote sensible, reliable, and efficient methods of research.

MRMC publications:

* *Perspectives on Animal Research*, volume 1, 1989

The contents include evaluation of learned helplessness research, physiological psychology research, head injury research on cats, amblyopia research on cats, Draize eye and skin tests, mathematical models, and use of animals in veterinary education. ($10; $5 for MRMC members)

* *Perspectives on Animal Research*, volume 1 supplement, 1989.

This special edition features a 134-page review of ten randomly chosen animal models of human diseases. ($10; $5 for MRMC members)

* *A Critical Look at Animal Research*

This pamphlet summarizes MRMC's concerns about the value of animal models. ($2.40; free for MRMC members)

MRMC Report -- quarterly newsletter (free to MRMC members)

MRMC membership is $25 per year, $10 for students and residents.